Better Homes and Gardens®

EATING WELL

With the
Food Guide Pyramid

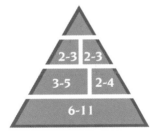

D0507590

BETTER HOMES AND GARDENS® BOOKS
Des Moines, Iowa

BETTER HOMES AND GARDENS® BOOKS
An Imprint of Meredith® Books

Eating Well with the Food Guide Pyramid
Editor: Kristi Fuller, R.D.
Copy Chief: Gregory H. Kayko
Associate Art Director: Lynda Haupert
Contributing Writer: Diane Quagliani, M.B.A., R.D.
Recipe Development: Linda Henry
Electronic Production Coordinator: Paula Forest
Test Kitchen Product Supervisor: Marilyn Cornelius
Illustrator: Steve Shock
Production Manager: Douglas Johnston

Director, New Product Development: Ray Wolf
Managing Editor: Christopher Cavanaugh
Test Kitchen Director: Sharon Stilwell

Meredith Publishing Group
President, Publishing Group: Christopher Little
Vice President and Publishing Director: John P. Loughlin

Meredith Corporation
Chairman of the Board and Chief Executive Officer: Jack D. Rehm
President and Chief Operating Officer: William T. Kerr

Chairman of the Executive Committee: E. T. Meredith III

All of us at Better Homes and Gardens® Books are dedicated to providing you with the information and ideas you need to create delicious foods. We welcome your comments and suggestions. Write to us at: Better Homes and Gardens® Books, Cookbook Editorial Department, RW-240, 1716 Locust St., Des Moines, IA 50309-3023

If you would like to order additional copies of any of our books, call 1-800-678-2803 or check with your local bookstore.

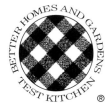

Our seal assures you that every recipe in *Eating Well with the Food Guide Pyramid* has been tested in the Better Homes and Gardens® Test Kitchen. This means that each recipe is practical and reliable, and meets our high standards of taste appeal. We guarantee your satisfaction with this book for as long as you own it.

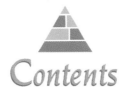

Contents

Eating Well

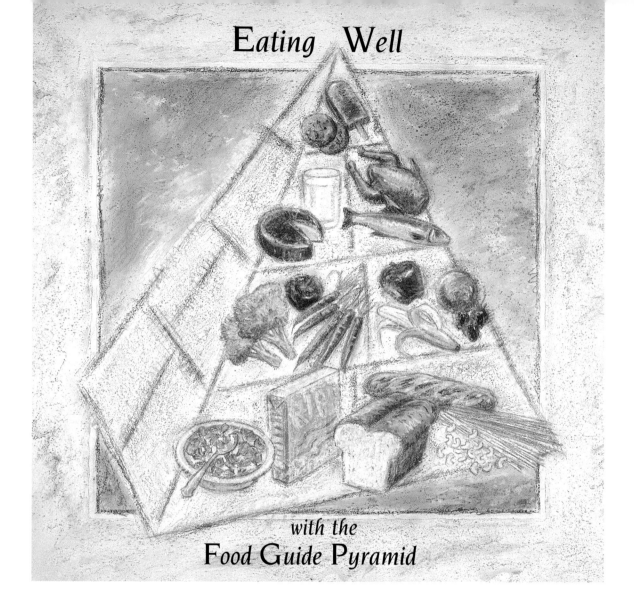

with the
Food Guide Pyramid

Thanks to the Food Guide Pyramid, you can enjoy your lifestyle—
and maintain a balanced diet, too.

▲ Is it possible to eat healthily while you're on the run?
▲ Can you provide your family members the nutrition they need?
▲ Can you enjoy a dessert and still eat well?

The answer to all of these questions is a hearty "yes." The Food Guide Pyramid stacks up as an easy-to-follow guide to good eating. This three-sided structure steers you past too much fat, saturated fat, cholesterol, sugar, and sodium and shows you how to meet important calorie and nutrition needs. Best of all, the Pyramid gives a green light to all your favorite foods.

In this book, you'll find dozens of recipes, tested by the **Better Homes and Gardens Test Kitchen,** to help you make the most of the Pyramid. There are no rigid calorie counts, no portions to weigh and measure—just common-sense guidelines for making balanced nutrition a habit in your daily life.

Using This Cookbook As Your Guide

This book makes the Pyramid easy to use by offering you page after page of healthful recipes. With each one, you will see at a glance the number of Pyramid food group servings you'll get in one serving of the recipe. In addition, the inside of the front cover and page 96 provide quick-and-easy reference information. We hope you'll refer to this book

The USDA Dietary Guidelines For Americans

Eat a variety of foods
Balance the food you eat with physical activity; maintain or improve your weight
Choose a diet with plenty of grain products, vegetables, and fruits
Choose a diet low in fat, saturated fat, and cholesterol
Choose a diet moderate in sugars
Choose a diet moderate in salt and sodium
If you drink alcoholic beverages, do so in moderation

often as you prepare nutritious, well-balanced meals, helping your entire family benefit from the Pyramid approach to eating. But, before you check out the recipes, let's scale the Pyramid to see how it will work for you.

Climbing the Food Guide Pyramid

The Food Guide Pyramid is a tool to good nutrition for healthy Americans ages two years old and up. Developed by the U.S. Department of Agriculture and the Department of Health and Human Services, the Pyramid represents the latest research-based nutrition advice.

Low-Fat Benefits

The risk of developing illnesses such as heart disease, high blood pressure, stroke, diabetes, and some cancers has been linked to eating too much fat—especially saturated fat. In addition to improving your diet, eating the Pyramid way helps you reduce the risk of developing these specific illnesses by trimming total fat from the foods you choose.

Bottom Line: The Food Guide Pyramid shows you how to put the Dietary Guidelines for Americans into practice.

The Pyramid is built from five food groups that fit together like a puzzle. Each group gives you some, but not all, of the nutrients your body needs. To make your own personal nutrition picture complete, choose foods from every group every day, and eat a variety of foods from within each of the groups.

How many daily servings should you eat from the Pyramid food groups? Because everyone has different calorie and nutrition needs, the Pyramid includes a range of servings in each group. While just about everyone should eat at least the minimum number of servings, the amount depends on the number of calories you need—and that depends on your age, sex, size, and level of daily activity. As a guideline, see the chart, *How Many Calories Do You Need*, page 9.

You can hit your calorie and fat targets by choosing lower-fat options in each food group and going easy on "extras," such as fats, oils, and sweets. The chart on the front inside cover shows the number of servings from each group recommended for three daily calorie levels, plus the fat grams.

The size of your servings is important, too, but don't worry about measuring and weighing your food! Consider the Pyramid serving sizes as general guidelines. Check page 96 for the serving sizes of various foods in each of the Pyramid groups.

How the Pyramid Stacks Up

To help you learn your way around the Pyramid, let's explore each food group in detail from the ground up.

Breads, Cereals, Rice, & Pasta

The base of the Pyramid represents the largest group. It contains foods made from grains, including breads, cereals, rice, pasta, breadsticks, pizza crust, crackers, pretzels, popcorn, pancakes, bagels, and more.

In the same way the Bread Group serves as the Pyramid's foundation, the foods in this group form the foundation for healthful eating—and it's no wonder. Naturally low in fat and high in energy-giving complex carbohydrates, they provide B-vitamins, vitamin E, iron, zinc, calcium, magnesium, and copper.

Whole grains, such as whole wheat bread, bran flakes, and brown rice, also provide valuable fiber.

From this food group, you need six to eleven servings a day. If that sounds like more than you can eat, keep in mind that the servings are modest. For example, a serving equals one slice of bread; an ounce of ready-to-eat cereal; or a half cup of cooked cereal, rice, or pasta. Your typical helping of pasta may count for two or three servings!

If you're worried about gaining weight from eating all those starchy foods, don't be. The real culprits are the fatty ingredients and toppings we pair them with—oil, butter, margarine, cheese, and rich sauces, just to name a few. Ounce for ounce, fats pack more than twice the calories of carbohydrate-rich grains. So, go light on the fat, dig into the Bread Group, and enjoy!

Vegetables

Moving up to the next level of the Pyramid, you'll find the Vegetable Group and its partner, the Fruit Group. A busy schedule is no reason to come up short on your daily quota. With an abundance of prewashed, ready-cut, and microwaveable veggies on the market, you can snack on baby carrots almost anywhere or toss up a salad in seconds.

Vegetables are a nutrition bargain, too. Low in calories and fat, they're bursting with vitamin C, folic acid, beta carotene, iron, magnesium, and fiber. To make the most of these nutrients, select a wide variety from the bounty at your supermarket. Several times a week, treat yourself to dark green, leafy vegetables, such as spinach, romaine lettuce, broccoli, or cabbage, and choose deep yellow and orange varieties, such as carrots, sweet potatoes, and acorn squash. Plan to eat at least three to five servings of vegetables each day. Refer to page 96 for serving equivalents.

Fruits

Fruits give you vitamin C, beta carotene, potassium, and fiber—all wrapped up in a sweet, fat-free package. And talk about fast food! Toss an apple or a mini box of raisins into your backpack or purse for a nutritious on-the-go snack.

The Pyramid suggests two to four servings of fruit each day. Super-nutritious choices include deep yellow or orange fruits (cantaloupe, apricots, peaches, or mangoes) and "high C" options (oranges, grapefruits, strawberries, or kiwi). To boost your fiber intake, opt for whole fruit more often than juices. See page 96 for serving equivalents.

Milk, Yogurt, & Cheese

On the next level of the Pyramid are Milk, Yogurt, and Cheese. The foods in this group supply approximately three-quarters of the calcium we consume, and they also provide protein, phosphorous, magnesium, and vitamins A, D, B_{12}, and riboflavin.

Though regular varieties of Milk Group foods often are high in fat (especially saturated fat), there are many low-fat and non-fat versions available. Smart selections include skim or 1 percent low-fat milk, fat-free or low-fat yogurt, and fat-free or reduced-fat cheese. Ice cream and frozen yogurt count here, too, but they often pack more of a calorie wallop. Save them for sweet treats, and select low-fat and fat-free types.

Most people need at least two daily servings from the Milk Group. Pregnant or breast-feeding women, teens, and young adults up to the age of 24 need three servings. See page 96 for serving equivalents of foods from this group.

Meat, Poultry, Fish, Dry Beans, Eggs, & Nuts

Next door to the Milk Group are Meat, Poultry, Fish, Dry Beans, Eggs, and Nuts. Foods in this group are important for good health because they contribute protein, B vitamins, iron, and zinc.

Meat Group: Sample Daily Servings

If your daily goal from the Meat Group is 6 ounces (2 to 3 servings), your choices might look like this:

Breakfast	
A scrambled egg	1 ounce
Lunch	
Soup with ½ cup of beans	1 ounce
Sandwich with 2 tablespoons peanut butter	1 ounce
Dinner	
Lean broiled steak	3 ounces
TOTAL:	6 ounces

Think lean when selecting foods from this group. Choose cuts of meat with the words "round" or "loin" in the name (e.g., ground round or pork tenderloin), skinless poultry, fish, and dry beans and peas.

Include two to three servings each day from the Meat Group, for a total of five to seven ounces. (See examples in chart *above*.) The chart on the inside of the front cover will help you determine the total number of ounces that are right for you.

As a general guideline, you can count two to three ounces of cooked lean meat, poultry, or fish as one serving. One ounce is about the size of a matchbox; three ounces is about the size of a deck of cards. See page 96 for serving equivalents.

The Tip of the Pyramid

Fats, oils, and sweets are grouped in the tip of the Pyramid. The tip is the smallest part of the Pyramid because most of us can afford to eat only small amounts of these foods. That's because they supply calories, but few, if any, vitamins or minerals. These foods include butter, margarine, oils, mayonnaise, salad dressing, cream, sugar, jam, jelly, soft drinks, candy, and most sweet desserts.

Serving sizes aren't provided for foods in the tip. Instead, remember to use them sparingly to enhance your enjoyment of foods from the five Pyramid food groups.

More Pyramid Pointers

The Pyramid can help you lose weight, enjoy your favorite foods, and eat a balanced diet—all at the same time. See page 10 for tips on how to make the most of the Pyramid.

How Many Calories Do You Need ?

The number of servings you need from each of the Pyramid food groups depends on age, sex, size, and level of activity. Follow the chart, below, and refer to the information on the inside of the front cover for the number of servings equivalent to specific calorie levels.

	Approximate Number of Calories Needed Daily
Preschoolers	Less than 1,600*
Children	2,200
Teenagers	
Girls	2,200
Boys	2,800
Women	
Sedentary	1,600
Active	2,200
Very active	2,800
(Pregnant or breast-feeding women may need more than 2,200.)	
Men	
Sedentary	2,200
Active	2,800
Older adults	1,600

*Though preschoolers require fewer calories, they need foods from all of the Pyramid food groups. Serve smaller portions, but make sure they have the equivalent of 2 cups of milk each day.

▲ **No Forbidden Foods.** If you think chocolate cake is off limits because it's not pictured in the Pyramid, think again. It fits in the Bread Group. That's because no foods are forbidden. The beauty of the Pyramid is that you can enjoy all of your favorite foods by balancing higher-fat choices with lower-fat ones and by keeping an eye on serving sizes. So team up a modest slice of your favorite chocolate cake with a tall glass of cold skim milk, then savor every bite!

▲ **Combination Foods.** Not everything you eat fits neatly into one food group. Do your best to divvy up "combination" foods. For example, for lasagna, you can assign the noodles to the Bread Group, tomato sauce to the Vegetable Group, cheese to the Milk Group, and ground beef to the Meat Group.

▲ **Fats and Sugars.** Throughout the Pyramid, there are fats and sugars found in all of the food groups. The fats are both added to and found naturally in foods; the sugar may be added sugar. Most of these sugars and fats are found in foods that fit into the Pyramid tip, followed by the Milk and Meat Groups. Although foods from the Bread, Vegetable, and Fruit Groups are naturally low in fat and added sugars, fats and sugars appear in those groups, too, because we sometimes choose such foods as buttered bread, French fries, or fruits canned in syrup.

▲ **A Pound of Prevention.** Let the Pyramid be your guide to shedding extra pounds and keeping them off. To lose weight, trim calories by eating the number of servings that's right for you from each Pyramid food group, but choose lower-fat and lower-sugar options. Go especially easy on alcohol and fats, oils, and sweets from the Pyramid tip. Once you reach your goal, it's OK to eat more of these foods, but only in small amounts. Also, remember the importance of physical activity for achieving a healthful weight, and always consult your physician before starting any exercise program.

▲ **A Drink or Two.** Alcohol, including beer, wine, and liquor, is not included in the Pyramid. Alcohol contains calories but has little nutritional value. If you're a healthy, non-pregnant adult and decide to drink, stick to one to two drinks a day—tops.

▲ **Easy Does It!** Falling a bit short on meeting Pyramid goals? The secret to success is making one small, easy change at a time. For instance, to cut back on fat, switch from regular mayonnaise to fat-free mayonnaise on your lunchtime sandwich; the following week, start snacking on pretzels instead of chips. Small changes like these add up to top nutrition over time.

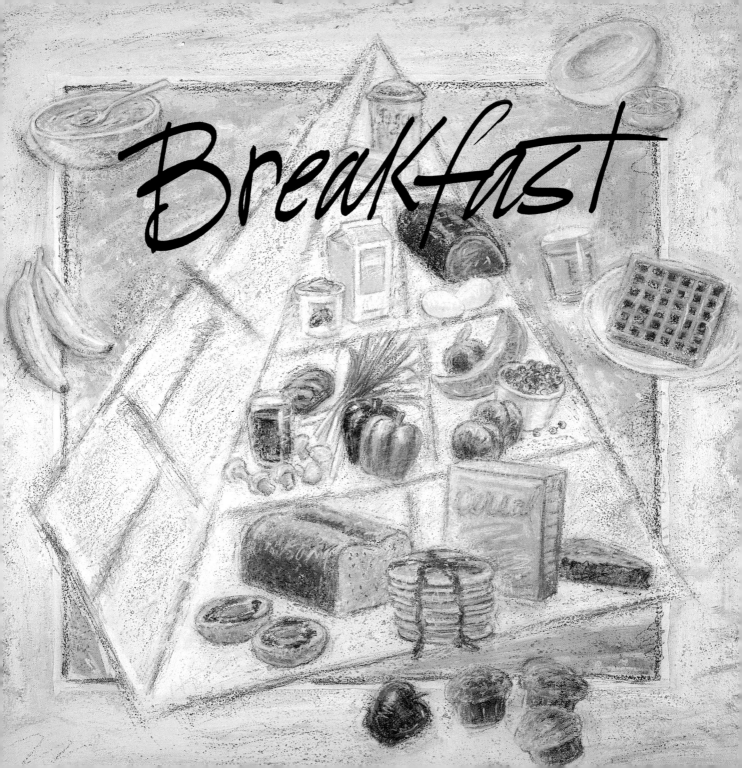

Breakfast

Breakfast Menus

Monday
Oatmeal with Dates and Nuts
   (page 13)
Fruit yogurt
Orange juice

Tuesday
Berry-Yogurt Drink (page 17)
Whole wheat toast
Margarine or butter
Spreadable fruit or jelly

Wednesday
Blueberry Muffins (page 18)
Mixed fresh fruit
Skim milk

Thursday
Waffley Good Sandwich
   (page 17)
Skim milk

Friday
Banana-Berry Muesli (page 20)
Toasted English muffin
Margarine or butter
Spreadable fruit or jelly
Skim milk

Saturday
Banana Stuffed French Toast
   (page 15)
Maple syrup
Turkey bacon
Skim milk

Sunday
Cheesy Grits and Sausage
   (page 16)
Melon wedges
Skim milk

Oatmeal with Dates and Nuts

1½ **cups water**
¼ **teaspoon ground cinnamon**
⅛ **teaspoon salt**
⅔ **cup regular rolled oats**
½ **small apple, cored and chopped**
2 **tablespoons snipped pitted dates**
1 **tablespoon toasted sliced almonds**
1½ **teaspoons brown sugar**
1⅓ **cups skim milk**

▲ In a medium saucepan combine the water, cinnamon, and salt. Bring to boiling; stir in the oats. Cook for 5 minutes, stirring occasionally. Let mixture stand, covered, till of desired consistency.

▲ Divide oatmeal mixture between 2 serving bowls. Top each serving of oatmeal with some chopped apple, snipped dates, sliced almonds, and brown sugar. Divide milk between each serving. Makes 2 servings.

Nutrition Facts per serving: 238 calories, 4 g total fat (1 g saturated fat), 3 mg cholesterol, 225 mg sodium, 42 g carbohydrate, 2 g fiber, 11 g protein.
Daily Values: 10% vitamin A, 5% vitamin C, 20% calcium, 11% iron.

Dates add a touch of natural sweetness to this cereal, but they also contribute fiber. Eat only a few at a time, though. They're a concentrated source of calories.

Oatmeal: Breakfast of Champs

Of course, oatmeal tastes great with a splash of milk and a little brown sugar. But it takes on a new personality with just a little creativity, as evidenced by this recipe. Aside from its versatility, oatmeal also has many nutritional virtues, such as several B vitamins, vitamin E, iron, and calcium. Oatmeal, or rolled oats, also contains a high amount of protein and is blessed with soluble fiber, a type of fiber that helps reduce blood cholesterol. Oats also make a tasty addition to breads, rolls, muffins, cookies, pancakes, waffles, or fruit desserts.

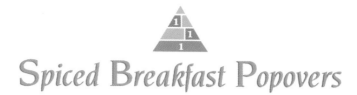

Spiced Breakfast Popovers

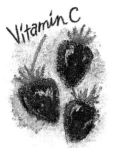
Vitamin C

Sweet and sensational, the strawberries in one serving of this luscious breakfast supply 75% of your vitamin C needs for the day.

Orange Cream
Nonstick spray coating
1 **beaten egg**
2 **slightly beaten egg whites**
1 **cup skim milk**
1 **tablespoon cooking oil**
1 **cup all-purpose flour**
⅛ **teaspoon salt**
3 **cups halved or quartered fresh strawberries**
Powdered sugar

▲ Prepare Orange Cream; cover and refrigerate till serving time. For popovers, generously spray nonstick coating on the insides of a popover pan; set aside.

▲ In a medium mixing bowl use a wire whisk or a rotary beater to beat together the whole egg, egg whites, milk, and oil. Add flour and salt. Beat with a rotary beater or a whisk till mixture is smooth. Fill prepared cups *half* full with batter. Bake in a 400° oven about 35 minutes or till popovers are firm.

▲ Remove popovers from oven and immediately prick each one with the tines of a fork to let the steam escape. Turn off the oven. (For crisper popovers, return popovers to the oven for 5 to 10 minutes or till desired crispness is reached.)

▲ Remove popovers from cups. To serve, split warm popovers in half crosswise and top with Orange Cream and strawberries. Sprinkle powdered sugar over each serving. Makes 6 servings.

Orange Cream: In a small mixing bowl combine 1½ cups *fat-free dairy sour cream*, 3 tablespoons *brown sugar*, ½ teaspoon finely shredded *orange peel*, 2 tablespoons *orange juice*, and ¼ teaspoon ground *cinnamon*. Cover and chill up to 24 hours.

Nutrition Facts per serving: 233 calories, 4 g total fat (1 g saturated fat), 36 mg cholesterol, 137 mg sodium, 39 g carbohydrate, 2 g fiber, 10 g protein.
Daily Values: 12% vitamin A, 75% vitamin C, 14% calcium, 9% iron.

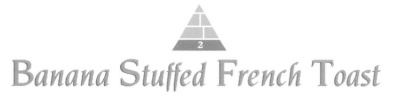

Banana Stuffed French Toast

Nonstick spray coating
1 **beaten egg**
1 **slightly beaten egg white**
½ **cup skim milk**
½ **teaspoon vanilla**
⅛ **teaspoon ground cinnamon**
6 **1-inch-thick slices French bread**
1 **medium banana, thinly sliced**
¼ **cup coconut, toasted**
   **Sifted powdered sugar, light
   pancake syrup product, or
   maple syrup (optional)**

▲ Spray a baking sheet with nonstick coating. In a shallow bowl beat together egg, egg white, milk, vanilla, and cinnamon. Set baking sheet and egg mixture aside.

▲ Using a knife, cut a pocket horizontally in each slice of bread cutting from the top crust almost to the bottom crust. Fill *each* bread pocket with *some* of the banana and coconut.

▲ Dip bread into egg mixture, coating both sides. Place bread on prepared baking sheet. Bake in a 500° oven for 5 minutes. Turn and bake for 5 to 6 minutes more or till golden brown. If desired, sprinkle with powdered sugar or serve with warm syrup. Makes 6 servings.

Nutrition Facts per serving: 183 calories, 4 g total fat (1 g saturated fat), 36 mg cholesterol, 295 mg sodium, 31 g carbohydrate, 0 g fiber, 6 g protein.
Daily Values: 2% vitamin A, 3% vitamin C, 5% calcium, 8% iron.

This scrumptious breakfast supplies two servings from the Bread Group of the Pyramid— a third of the recommended six servings per day.

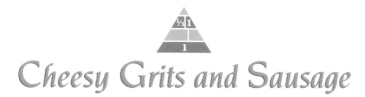

Cheesy Grits and Sausage

Grits, a high-carbohydrate cereal with a Southern tradition, comes from dried, hulled, and ground corn kernels. Quick-cooking grits save you time in this tasty breakfast dish.

4 cups water
1 cup quick-cooking grits
1 cup refrigerated or frozen egg product, thawed, or 4 beaten eggs
1 cup shredded reduced-fat cheddar cheese (4 ounces)
8 ounces turkey breakfast sausage, cooked and drained
¼ cup sliced green onion
1 to 2 fresh jalapeño peppers, seeded and finely chopped
½ teaspoon garlic salt
⅛ teaspoon ground black pepper
    Nonstick spray coating
2 tablespoons snipped parsley

▲ In a 2- or 3-quart saucepan bring water to boiling. Slowly add grits, stirring constantly. Bring to boiling. Reduce heat; cook and stir for 6 to 7 minutes or till the water is absorbed and mixture is thickened.

▲ Gradually stir about ½ cup grits mixture into egg product. Return egg-and-grits mixture to saucepan. Add ½ cup of the cheese to grits, stirring till cheese is melted. Stir in the cooked and drained turkey sausage, green onion, jalapeño peppers, garlic salt, and black pepper.

▲ Spray a 2-quart-rectangular baking dish with nonstick coating; spoon the grits mixture into baking dish.

▲ Bake in a 325° oven for 25 to 30 minutes or till set in the center. Sprinkle with remaining ½ cup cheese and parsley. Let stand for 5 minutes before serving. Makes 8 servings.

Nutrition Facts per serving: 203 calories, 7 g total fat (3 g saturated fat), 21 mg cholesterol, 505 mg sodium, 17 g carbohydrate, 0 g fiber, 16 g protein.
Daily Values: 10% vitamin A, 12% vitamin C, 10% calcium, 13% iron.

Easy Breakfast Ideas

Morning Shake:
In a blender container combine ½ cup orange juice, ½ cup vanilla low-fat yogurt, and 1 frozen banana. Cover and blend till smooth. Serves 1.

Apple-icious Oatmeal
Prepare a single serving of oatmeal according to package directions, *except* substitute apple juice for half of the water. Stir in ¼ cup chopped apple and a spoonful of maple syrup or pancake syrup. Serves 1.

X-tra Easy Oatmeal Muffins
Combine 1 slightly beaten egg, ⅔ cup reduced-fat biscuit mix, 1 envelope instant oatmeal with apples and cinnamon, and ⅓ cup skim milk. Fill 6 greased muffin cups ⅔ full. Bake in a 375° oven 18 to 20 minutes. Serves 6.

Berry Breakfast Parfaits
In parfait glasses, alternate layers of your favorite berry-flavored low-fat yogurt and fresh raspberries, blueberries, blackberries, or strawberries. Top with low-fat granola. Serves 1.

Berry-Yogurt Drink
In a blender container combine ½ cup frozen blueberries or strawberries, ½ cup vanilla low-fat yogurt, ¼ cup skim milk, and 1 tablespoon toasted wheat germ. Cover and blend till smooth. Serves 1.

Waffley Good Sandwich
Toast 2 frozen waffles according to package directions. Spread 1 waffle with 1 tablespoon reduced-fat peanut butter. Arrange 1 small banana, sliced, on top of peanut butter. Top with second warm waffle. Cut in half. Serves 1.

Just Peachy Drink
In a blender container combine one undrained 8¼-ounce can peach slices (juice pack), ¼ cup nonfat dry milk powder, ¼ cup orange juice or pineapple-orange juice, and ¼ teaspoon ground cinnamon. Cover and blend till smooth. With blender running, add 4 or 5 ice cubes, 1 at a time, through opening in lid. Pour into glasses. Serves 2.

Breakfast Burrito
In a small microwave-safe bowl stir together 1 egg, 2 egg whites, 2 tablespoons shredded reduced-fat sharp cheddar cheese, and 1 tablespoon skim milk. Micro-cook on high 1½ to 2 minutes, stirring every 30 seconds. Roll up in a warm flour tortilla and top with salsa. Serves 1.

Fruity Rolls
Spread ½ cup low-calorie fruit spread (such as apple raspberry) in a 9x1½-inch round baking pan. Separate one 11-ounce package (8) refrigerated breadsticks (do not uncoil) and place rolls atop fruit spread. Bake in a 375° oven for 15 to 18 minutes or till golden. Immediately invert onto a platter. Serve warm. Serves 8.

Grain and Fruit Cereal
Combine 1 cup cornmeal, ⅔ cup bulgur, a 6-ounce package chopped mixed dried fruit bits, ½ cup toasted slivered almonds, and ½ teaspoon ground cinnamon. Store cereal mixture in an airtight container. Makes enough for 8 servings.

For 1 serving, bring 1 cup water to boiling. Stir in ⅓ *cup* of the mixture. Simmer, uncovered, stirring occasionally, for 10 to 15 minutes. Serve with skim milk.

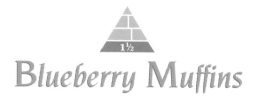

Blueberry Muffins

On days when you want something special for breakfast, muffins are an excellent substitute for toast. These count as 1½ servings from the Pyramid Bread Group.

Nonstick spray coating
1¾ **cups all-purpose flour**
⅓ **cup sugar**
2 **teaspoons baking powder**
⅛ **teaspoon salt**
1 **slightly beaten egg white**
¾ **cup skim milk**
3 **tablespoons cooking oil**
1 **teaspoon finely shredded orange peel**
1 **tablespoon orange juice**
¾ **cup fresh or frozen blueberries**
1 **to 2 teaspoons sugar**

▲ Spray twelve 2½-inch muffin cups with nonstick coating; set aside.

▲ In a medium mixing bowl stir together the flour, the ⅓ cup sugar, baking powder, and salt. Make a well in the center.

▲ In another mixing bowl stir together the egg white, milk, cooking oil, orange peel, and orange juice. Add all at once to the flour mixture. Stir just till mixture is moistened but still slightly lumpy. Gently fold in blueberries. Fill prepared muffin cups ⅔ full. Sprinkle lightly with the additional sugar.

▲ Bake in a 375° oven for 20 to 25 minutes or till tops are golden. Remove muffins from pans. Cool slightly on a wire rack. Serve warm. Makes 12 muffins.

Nutrition Facts per muffin: 125 calories, 4 g total fat (1 g saturated fat), 0 mg cholesterol, 84 mg sodium, 21 g carbohydrate, 1 g fiber, 3 g protein.
Daily Values: 1% vitamin A, 4% vitamin C, 7% calcium, 5% iron.

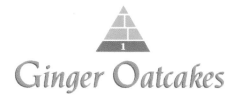

Ginger Oatcakes

1½ cups skim milk
¾ cup quick-cooking or regular
rolled oats
1 cup all-purpose flour
2 tablespoons finely chopped
crystallized ginger or ¼ to
½ teaspoon ground ginger
1½ teaspoons baking powder
¾ teaspoon ground cinnamon
¼ teaspoon baking soda
¼ teaspoon salt
3 beaten egg whites
1 beaten egg
2 tablespoons cooking oil
2 tablespoons dark corn syrup or
molasses
Fresh blueberries or sliced
banana (optional)
Orange marmalade or maple
syrup (optional)

▲ In a medium saucepan heat milk over low heat just till hot, stirring occasionally. Stir in the oats. Remove from heat; let stand 5 minutes. Combine flour, ginger, baking powder, cinnamon, baking soda, and salt; stir into oat mixture. Combine the egg whites, whole egg, cooking oil, and corn syrup; stir into oat mixture. Add oat mixture to flour mixture; stir till moistened. (Pancake batter may be covered and stored in the refrigerator for up to 2 days.)

▲ For *each* pancake, pour a scant *¼ cup* batter onto a hot, lightly greased heavy skillet. Cook till golden brown, turning to cook other side when surface is bubbly with slightly dry edges. If desired, serve pancakes topped with blueberries or sliced bananas and orange marmalade or maple syrup. Makes 14 pancakes.

Nutrition Facts per pancake: 94 calories, 3 g total fat (0 g saturated fat), 16 mg cholesterol, 132 mg sodium, 14 g carbohydrate, 1 g fiber, 4 g protein.
Daily Values: 2% vitamin A, 0% vitamin C, 6% calcium, 5% iron.

Top each serving of pancakes with a half cup of blueberries or one small sliced banana to supply a serving from the Pyramid Fruit Group.

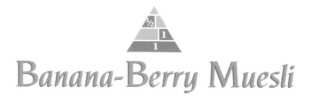

Banana-Berry Muesli

Muesli (MYOOS-lee), which means mixture in German, is a healthful breakfast cereal. Rolled oats and dried fruit are both good sources of fiber.

⅓ **cup regular rolled oats**
1 **8-ounce carton blueberry or spiced apple low-fat yogurt**
¾ **cup low-fat granola (purchased or homemade, see below)**
1 **medium banana, sliced**
⅓ **cup raisins, snipped apricots, or dried fruit bits**
1 **cup skim milk**

▲ Cook oats according to package directions. To serve, stir blueberry or apple yogurt into warm oatmeal. Reserve ¼ *cup* of the granola for the topping; set aside.

▲ Fold remaining granola, banana, and raisins or dried fruit into the yogurt-oatmeal mixture. Spoon the mixture into 4 cereal bowls. Top *each* serving with 1 *tablespoon* of the reserved granola. Serve with milk. Makes 4 servings.

Nutrition Facts per serving: 229 calories, 2 g total fat (1 g saturated fat), 3 mg cholesterol, 86 mg sodium, 47 g carbohydrate, 2 g fiber, 7 g protein.
Daily Values: 13% vitamin A, 6% vitamin C, 14% calcium, 10% iron.

Homemade Granola

To make your own granola, in a medium bowl combine 1½ cups *regular rolled oats*, ½ cup shredded unpeeled *apple*, and ¼ cup toasted *wheat germ*; set aside. In a small saucepan combine 2 tablespoons *honey*, 2 tablespoons *water*, and ½ teaspoon ground *cinnamon*. Heat to boiling; remove from heat. Stir in 1 teaspoon *vanilla*. Pour over oat mixture, tossing to coat. Spray a 15x10x1-inch baking pan with *nonstick spray coating*. Spread oat mixture in pan. Bake mixture in a 325° oven about 45 minutes or till golden brown, stirring occasionally. Spread onto foil to cool. Store granola in an airtight container in the refrigerator for up to 2 weeks. Makes four ½-cup servings.

Calories: 179 Total Fat: 3 grams

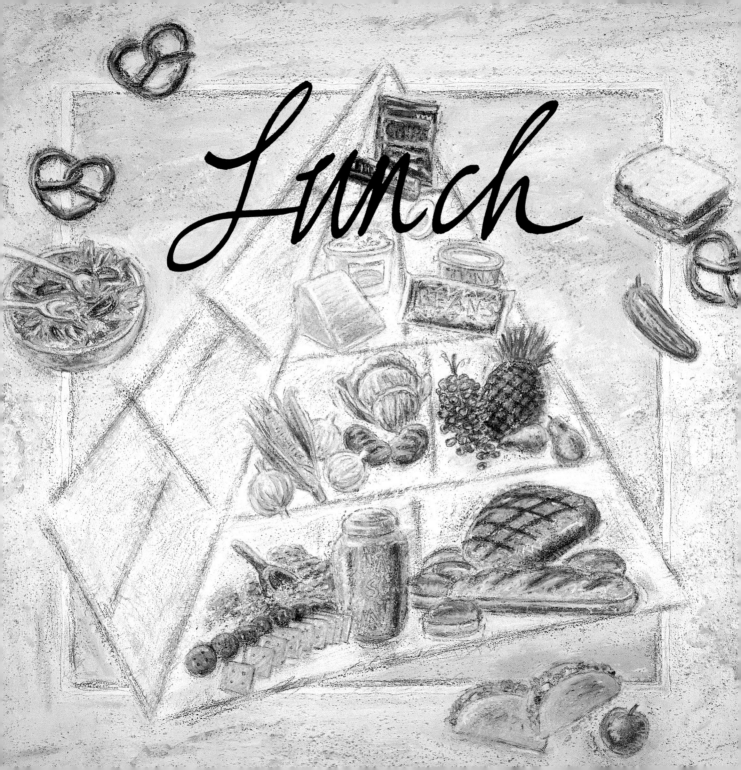

Lunch Menus

Monday
Dilled Veggie and Cheese
   Sandwiches (page 30)
Pretzels
Bean soup
Sparkling water

Tuesday
Tortilla and Blue Cheese
   Roll-up (page 25)
Baked Tortilla Chips (page 86)
Apple
Skim milk

Wednesday
Chicken Salad with Avocado
   Dressing (page 34)
Whole-grain crackers
Skim milk

Thursday
Chicken Tabbouleh (page 41)
Pita bread
Grapes
Skim milk

Friday
Cajun Fish Sandwiches with
   Slaw (page 23)
Rye crackers
Pear
Skim milk

Saturday
Potato Corn Chowder (page 39)
Sliced fresh tomatoes
Low-fat vinaigrette
Whole-grain roll
Sparkling water

Sunday
Snappy Joes (page 27)
Baked potato fries
Mixed greens salad
Low-fat salad dressing
Skim milk

Cajun Fish Sandwiches with Slaw

1½ cups packaged shredded
    cabbage with carrot
    (cole slaw mix)
  2 tablespoons reduced-calorie
    mayonnaise dressing or salad
    dressing
    Dash Cajun seasoning
12 ounces fresh or frozen catfish
    fillets, about ½ inch thick
  1 to 2 teaspoons Cajun seasoning
    Nonstick spray coating
  4 whole wheat hamburger buns,
    split and toasted

▲ For slaw, in a medium mixing bowl combine shredded cabbage, mayonnaise or salad dressing, and dash Cajun seasoning. Cover and chill till needed.

▲ Thaw fish, if frozen. Cut fish into 4 equal portions. Rinse and pat dry. Sprinkle the 1 to 2 teaspoons Cajun seasoning over both sides of fish. Spray a cold large nonstick skillet with nonstick coating. Preheat over medium heat. Cook fillets in hot skillet for 6 to 8 minutes or till fish begins to flake easily when tested with a fork, turning fish halfway through cooking. Serve fish on buns; top each with some of the slaw mixture. Makes 4 servings.

Nutrition Facts per serving: 273 calories, 11 g total fat (2 g saturated fat), 49 mg cholesterol, 375 mg sodium, 24 g carbohydrate, 2 g fiber, 18 g protein.
Daily Values: 23% vitamin A, 24% vitamin C, 4% calcium, 13% iron.

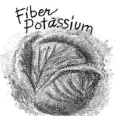

Fiber Potassium

As an added bonus, cabbage lends crunch, vitamin C, fiber, and potassium to this fish sandwich. Fish is high in omega-3 fatty acids, which help fight heart disease.

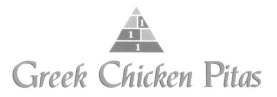

Greek Chicken Pitas

Popeye thought spinach was good for him. He was right—it is high in beta carotene, fiber, potassium, and iron. It's also a boon to calorie-watchers at only 40 calories per cup of fresh leaves. Add it liberally to this sandwich.

2 tablespoons skim milk
3 tablespoons fine dry bread crumbs
½ teaspoon dried oregano, crushed
½ teaspoon ground cumin
¼ teaspoon garlic salt
¼ teaspoon pepper
12 ounces ground raw chicken or turkey
½ cup plain nonfat yogurt
1 small cucumber, seeded and chopped
1 green onion, thinly sliced
2 teaspoons snipped fresh mint or ½ teaspoon dried mint, crushed
⅛ teaspoon sugar
2 large pita bread rounds, halved crosswise
1 cup shredded fresh spinach or lettuce

▲ In a medium mixing bowl combine milk, bread crumbs, oregano, cumin, garlic salt, and pepper. Add ground chicken or turkey; mix well. Form into 4 oval patties about ½ inch thick.

▲ Place patties on the unheated rack of a broiler pan. Broil 4 to 5 inches from the heat for 5 minutes. Turn over and broil for 5 to 10 minutes more or till chicken is no longer pink.

▲ Meanwhile, in a small bowl stir together yogurt, chopped cucumber, green onion, mint, and sugar.

▲ Split open each pita half, forming a pocket. Place some of the spinach or lettuce and a chicken patty in the pocket; top with yogurt mixture and remaining spinach. Makes 4 servings.

Nutrition Facts per serving: 177 calories, 5 g total fat (1 g saturated fat), 41 mg cholesterol, 326 mg sodium, 16 g carbohydrate, 1 g fiber, 17 g protein.
Daily Values: 11% vitamin A, 11% vitamin C, 9% calcium, 13% iron.

Sandwich Ideas

New PBJ

Combine 2 spoonfuls reduced-fat peanut butter, 1 spoonful apricot spreadable fruit, and a dash or two dry mustard. Spread onto a slice of raisin bread. Top with lettuce leaves, some thinly sliced apple, and a slice of raisin bread. Serves 1.

Tortilla and Blue Cheese Roll-up

Spread some blue cheese nonfat salad dressing onto 1 flour tortilla. Top with a lettuce leaf, 2 thin slices cooked beef, and a slice reduced-fat Swiss cheese. Roll up tightly. Serves 1.

Chicken Salad and Chutney

Prepare your favorite chicken salad recipe using nonfat mayonnaise dressing or salad dressing. Stir in a couple of spoonfuls halved seedless red grapes, a spoonful snipped chutney, and a dash curry powder. Serve on rye bread. Serves 1.

Spiced Turkey

Spread 2 slices of cinnamon-raisin bread with a spoonful orange low-fat yogurt. Top 1 slice with thinly sliced fully cooked smoked turkey breast, a lettuce leaf, and remaining bread slice. Serves 1.

Italian Tuna

Combine a 3-ounce can tuna (water-packed), drained; 2 spoonfuls low-calorie creamy Italian salad dressing; and 1/3 cup finely chopped seeded cucumber. Spoon into a lettuce-lined pita bread half. Serves 2.

Ham-and-Cheese

Combine a 5-ounce can chunk-style ham, drained and flaked, with 1/2 cup finely chopped mixed fresh vegetables, such as broccoli and/or green sweet pepper. Stir in 2 spoonfuls fat-free cream cheese. Line 3 pita bread halves with lettuce leaves. Spoon ham mixture into a pita halves. Serves 3.

Cranberry-Turkey

Combine one 5-ounce can chunk-style turkey (water-packed), drained and flaked, a few spoonfuls cranberry-orange relish, 2 spoonfuls reduced-calorie mayonnaise dressing, and a small finely chopped apple. Spread on 2 slices rye bread. Top with shredded spinach and a bread slice. Serves 2.

Curried Pork

Stir together 1/4 cup reduced-calorie mayonnaise dressing or salad dressing and a couple dashes curry powder. Stir in 1/2 cup finely chopped cooked pork, a small shredded carrot, and a spoonful of light raisins. Spread onto 2 slices whole wheat bread; top each with bean sprouts or lettuce and another slice of bread. Serves 2.

Pork and Apple Butter

Combine 1/4 cup apple butter and 2 small spoonfuls coarse-grain mustard. Spread 2 slices of pumpernickel bread with apple butter mixture. Top with thinly sliced cooked pork, preshredded coleslaw mix, and thinly sliced apple. Top each with another slice of bread. Serves 2.

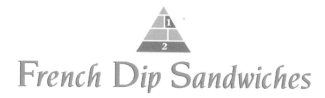

French Dip Sandwiches

Beef up your Bread Group servings with this classic lunch treat. The green pepper in the meat filling adds vitamin C, which helps boost the iron absorption from meat.

1¾ **cups water**
1 **small onion, sliced and separated into rings**
1 **small green sweet pepper, cored and sliced into rings**
2 **teaspoons Worcestershire sauce**
1 **teaspoon instant beef bouillon granules**
½ **teaspoon garlic powder**
⅛ **teaspoon pepper**
10 **ounces thinly sliced cooked beef**
4 **French-style rolls, split and toasted**

▲ In a medium saucepan combine the water, onion, green pepper, Worcestershire sauce, bouillon granules, garlic powder, and pepper. Bring to boiling. Reduce heat and simmer, covered, for 10 minutes. Add beef; return to boiling. Reduce heat and simmer, covered, about 5 minutes more or till heated.

▲ To serve, using a slotted spoon, spoon beef-and-vegetable mixture onto toasted rolls, reserving broth. Ladle reserved broth into 4 small bowls; serve with sandwiches for dipping. Makes 4 servings.

Nutrition Facts per serving: 278 calories, 9 g total fat (3 g saturated fat), 63 mg cholesterol, 522 mg sodium, 23 g carbohydrate, 0 g fiber, 26 g protein.
Daily Values: 0% vitamin A, 24% vitamin C, 4% calcium, 23% iron.

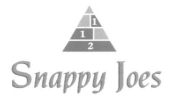

Snappy Joes

1 pound lean ground beef or
  ground raw turkey
½ cup chopped green sweet pepper
¼ cup chopped onion
1 8-ounce can tomato sauce
½ cup hot-style or regular bottled
  barbecue sauce
1 cup shredded cabbage with
  carrot (coleslaw mix)
8 whole wheat hamburger
  buns, split and toasted,
  or 8 baked potatoes

▲ In a large skillet cook the ground beef or turkey, green pepper, and onion for 4 to 5 minutes or till meat is no longer pink. Drain off fat. Stir in the tomato sauce, barbecue sauce, and cabbage with carrot. Bring to boiling; reduce heat. Simmer, uncovered, for 10 minutes.

▲ To serve, spoon some of the meat mixture into each bun or over each baked potato. Makes 8 servings.

Nutrition Facts per serving: 225 calories, 7 g total fat (2 g saturated fat), 36 mg cholesterol, 549 mg sodium, 27 g carbohydrate, 3 g fiber, 15 g protein.
Daily Values: 9% vitamin A, 21% vitamin C, 5% calcium, 16% iron.

To sneak a Vegetable Group serving into a quick lunch, add coleslaw mix to this flavorful sandwich. Look for the mix in the produce department of your supermarket. For variety, try the version made with broccoli.

Lean on Lower-Fat Beef

Cook with the leanest ground beef available to keep your low-fat goals in check. Look for 90 percent lean (10 percent fat). Some supermarkets offer 95 percent lean ground beef. This type of ground beef has some of the fat replaced with water and plant derivatives. Use lean ground beef in burgers, chili, tacos, or casseroles.

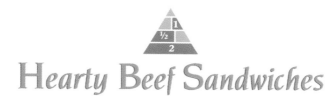

Hearty Beef Sandwiches

A simple sandwich can pack a lot of punch when it comes to meeting Pyramid serving recommendations. This tasty combo contributes two servings from the Bread Group, plus one from the Meat Group and a half serving from the Vegetable Group.

½ **cup fat-free dairy sour cream**
¼ **cup unsweetened applesauce**
2 **tablespoons prepared horseradish**
½ **teaspoon cracked pepper**
8 **slices marbled-rye, rye, or pumpernickel bread**
4 **lettuce leaves**
½ **cup canned beet slices, well drained**
6 **ounces thinly sliced cooked beef or one 6-ounce package very thinly sliced fully cooked beef**

▲ In a small mixing bowl combine the sour cream, applesauce, horseradish, and pepper. Spread about 1 *tablespoon* sour cream mixture onto *each* slice of bread.

▲ Place a lettuce leaf on each of 4 bread slices. Top with some beet slices and beef. Top with remaining bread slices, spread side down. Makes 4 servings.

Nutrition Facts per serving: 321 calories, 8 g total fat (3 g saturated fat), 34 mg cholesterol, 642 mg sodium, 41 g carbohydrate, 1 g fiber, 20 g protein.
Daily Values: 4% vitamin A, 8% vitamin C, 9% calcium, 25% iron.

Have a Safe Lunch

Keep your sandwich safe by following these tips:
▲ Seal foods in clean airtight containers or plastic storage bags. Chill cold foods overnight. Then, in the morning, pack them in prechilled* insulated vacuum containers or in insulated lunch boxes with frozen ice packs.
▲ Keep your lunch in a cool, dry place all morning. (Not in hot, stuffy cars or on sunny window ledges.)
   *Note: To prechill (or preheat) your insulated vacuum bottle, fill the bottle with the coldest (or hottest) tap water possible. Cover with the lid; let stand for 5 minutes. Empty the bottle, shaking out the excess water. Immediately fill the bottle with the cold (or hot) food.

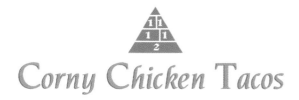

Corny Chicken Tacos

2 teaspoons chili powder
¼ teaspoon ground cumin
⅛ teaspoon salt
⅛ teaspoon onion powder
⅛ teaspoon ground red pepper
    (optional)
10 ounces skinless, boneless chicken
    breasts, cut into thin, bite-size
    strips
2 teaspoons cooking oil
1 cup loose-pack frozen whole
    kernel corn
8 taco shells
1 cup shredded lettuce
1 cup chopped tomato
½ cup shredded reduced-fat
    cheddar cheese (2 ounces)

▲ In a medium mixing bowl stir together the chili powder, cumin, salt, onion powder, and red pepper, if desired. Add the chicken and toss to coat. In a large skillet heat oil over medium-high heat. Add chicken and cook and stir about 3 minutes or till tender and no pink remains. Stir in corn; heat through.

▲ Meanwhile, warm the taco shells according to package directions. Fill each taco shell with some of the chicken-corn mixture. Top with lettuce, chopped tomato, and cheese. Makes 4 servings.

Nutrition Facts per serving: 298 calories, 12 g total fat (3 g saturated fat), 47 mg cholesterol, 315 mg sodium, 27 g carbohydrate, 1 g fiber, 21 g protein.
Daily Values: 10% vitamin A, 14% vitamin C, 13% calcium, 12% iron.

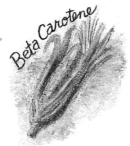

Although the health benefits attributed to beta carotene may entice you to take a supplement, the best advice is to eat foods rich in beta carotene. Its anti-cancer effect may be due to some other substance in these foods. Beta carotene is found only in plant foods, such as corn, tomatoes, and dark green or orange vegetables.

Dilled Veggie and Cheese Sandwiches

Foods from the Pyramid Milk Group are top sources for vitamins A, B_{12}, D, and riboflavin—all necessary nutrients in your diet. When selecting foods from this group, search out those that are lowest in fat and saturated fat, such as the ones used in this recipe.

½ of an 8-ounce package (4 ounces) fat-free cream cheese
2 tablespoons plain fat-free or low-fat yogurt
2 tablespoons snipped fresh dill or 1½ teaspoons dried dillweed
⅛ teaspoon pepper
8 slices multi-grain bread
4 fresh spinach leaves
4 ounces thinly sliced reduced-fat cheddar cheese
1 cup thinly sliced cucumber
1 tomato, thinly sliced
1 cup alfalfa sprouts

▲ In a small mixing bowl stir together cream cheese and yogurt till smooth; stir in dill and pepper. Spread 1 side of each bread slice with cream cheese mixture. Top 4 slices of bread with spinach leaves, cheddar cheese, cucumber slices, tomato slices, and alfalfa sprouts. Cover with remaining bread slices, spread side down. Makes 4 servings.

Nutrition Facts per serving: 262 calories, 7 g total fat (3 g saturated fat), 25 mg cholesterol, 467 mg sodium, 30 g carbohydrate, 1 g fiber, 19 g protein.
Daily Values: 20% vitamin A, 6% vitamin C, 30% calcium, 14% iron.

I'd Like Some Cheese, Please

To help hold down the fat, look for lower-fat and nonfat natural and processed cheeses. Here are some to consider:
▲ Reduced-fat natural cheese—A natural cheese, such as cheddar, Swiss, and Monterey Jack cheese, with fewer grams of fat than regular natural cheese. Lower-fat mozzarella is called "part-skim mozzarella cheese."
▲ Lower-fat flavored process cheese product—A lower-fat process cheese that is available in American, cheddar, or Swiss flavors.
▲ Nonfat process cheese product—A process cheese without any fat.

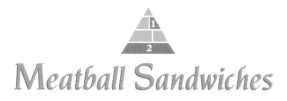

Meatball Sandwiches

4 individual loaves French bread (baguettes)
1 slightly beaten egg white
2 tablespoons finely chopped onion
1 teaspoon dried Italian seasoning, crushed
¼ teaspoon fennel seed, crushed
⅛ teaspoon salt
⅛ teaspoon ground red pepper
8 ounces lean ground beef
   Nonstick spray coating
1 cup sliced fresh mushrooms
1 small onion, chopped
2 cloves garlic, minced
1 14½-ounce can whole Italian-style tomatoes, cut up
2 tablespoons tomato paste
¼ teaspoon sugar
⅛ teaspoon pepper
   Shredded reduced-fat mozzarella cheese (optional)

▲ Cut a thin slice from top of each baguette. Scoop out bread from the bottom half of each loaf, leaving a ½-inch-thick shell. Set shells and tops aside. Place bread pieces in a food processor bowl or blender container. Cover; process or blend to soft bread crumbs. Measure ½ cup (reserve remaining crumbs for another use).

▲ For meatballs, in a mixing bowl stir together the ½ cup bread crumbs, egg white, the 2 tablespoons onion, ¼ *teaspoon* of the Italian seasoning, the fennel seed, salt, and red pepper. Add beef; mix well. Shape into 16 balls. Place meatballs in a 2-quart-square baking dish. Bake, uncovered, in a 375° oven about 20 minutes or till juices run clear. Drain off fat.

▲ For sauce, spray a cold medium saucepan with nonstick coating. Preheat pan over medium heat. Cook the mushrooms, chopped onion, and garlic for 2 to 3 minutes or till tender. Stir in *undrained* tomatoes, tomato paste, remaining Italian seasoning, sugar, and pepper. Bring to boiling; reduce heat. Simmer, uncovered, 5 to 10 minutes or to desired consistency.

▲ Gently stir meatballs into sauce. Spoon meatballs and sauce into rolls. If desired, top with cheese. Makes 4 servings.

Nutrition Facts per serving: 249 calories, 8 g total fat (3 g saturated fat), 36 mg cholesterol, 508 mg sodium, 30 g carbohydrate, 2 g fiber, 16 g protein.
Daily Values: 8% vitamin A, 36% vitamin C, 7% calcium, 23% iron.

What a treat— meatballs simmered in tomato sauce and served inside a French roll fulfill part of your bread and meat require- ments for the day. Add a little cheese to your sandwich to up your calcium intake.

Seafarer's Burgers & Cucumber Sauce

For a refreshing switch from mayonnaise, we've topped this fish sandwich with a blend of nonfat yogurt and shredded cucumber. Try shredded zucchini or carrots for other colorful alternatives.

1 **slightly beaten egg white**
¼ **cup fine dry bread crumbs**
¼ **cup shredded cucumber or zucchini**
2 **tablespoons nonfat mayonnaise dressing or salad dressing**
2 **teaspoons Dijon-style mustard**
2 **6-ounce cans crabmeat, drained, flaked, and cartilage removed, or two 6½-ounce cans tuna (water-packed), drained and flaked**
2 **tablespoons fine dry bread crumbs**
2 **tablespoons cornmeal**
4 **lettuce leaves**
4 **English muffins, split and toasted Cucumber Sauce**

▲ In a medium mixing bowl stir together egg white, the ¼ cup bread crumbs, cucumber or zucchini, mayonnaise or salad dressing, and mustard. Stir in crabmeat or tuna; mix well. Shape into 4 patties about ¾ inch thick.

▲ Combine remaining 2 tablespoons bread crumbs and cornmeal; coat patties with cornmeal mixture. Place on an ungreased baking sheet. Bake in a 450° oven for 12 to 15 minutes or till golden, turning once. Place a lettuce leaf on the bottom half of each muffin. Top with fish, Cucumber Sauce, and muffin tops. Makes 4 servings.

Cucumber Sauce: In a small mixing bowl combine ¼ cup shredded *cucumber*, ¼ cup *plain nonfat yogurt*, and ¼ teaspoon dried *dillweed*. Cover and refrigerate for up to 4 hours.

Nutrition Facts per serving: 297 calories, 3 g total fat (0 g saturated fat), 76 mg cholesterol, 802 mg sodium, 40 g carbohydrate, 1 g fiber, 26 g protein.
Daily Values: 1% vitamin A, 6% vitamin C, 19% calcium, 18% iron.

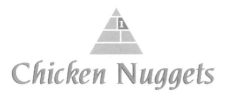

Chicken Nuggets

¾ **cup fine cornflake crumbs or**
   fine dry bread crumbs
1 **teaspoon paprika**
½ **teaspoon garlic powder**
½ **teaspoon dried oregano, crushed**
⅛ **teaspoon ground red pepper**
1 **slightly beaten egg white**
1 **pound skinless, boneless chicken**
   breast halves, cut into 1-inch
   pieces
   Honey-Mustard Sauce

▲ In a plastic bag combine cornflake or bread crumbs, paprika, garlic powder, oregano, and red pepper. Place egg white in a small bowl.

▲ Dip chicken pieces in egg white, allowing excess to drain off. Add pieces, a few at a time, to plastic bag. Close bag; shake to coat pieces well.

▲ Place pieces in a single layer in a 15x10x1-inch baking pan. Bake in a 450° oven for 7 to 9 minutes or till no longer pink. Serve with Honey-Mustard Sauce. Makes 4 servings.

Honey-Mustard Sauce: In a bowl stir together 2 tablespoons *prepared mustard* and 1 tablespoon *honey*.

Nutrition Facts per serving: 185 calories, 3 g total fat (1 g saturated fat), 59 mg cholesterol, 271 mg sodium, 12 g carbohydrate, 0 g fiber, 23 g protein.
Daily Values: 15% vitamin A, 8% vitamin C, 1% calcium, 10% iron.

A *single chicken nugget from your favorite fast food restaurant may contain as much fat as an entire serving of this baked version. Make your own at home and enjoy them guilt-free.*

Safety Points for Poultry

To keep poultry safe:
▲ Never leave cooked poultry at room temperature for more than 2 hours. Cover and refrigerate it as soon as possible.
▲ Always cook it thoroughly before eating. Poultry is done when the meat is no longer pink and the juices run clear.
▲ Wash your hands, counter, and utensils in hot, soapy water when handling or cutting up poultry.

Chicken Salad with Avocado Dressing

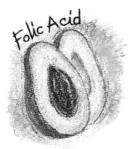
Folic Acid

It's true. California avocados contain quite a lot of fat and, thus, calories. But, fortunately, the fat is highly unsaturated. Avocados fare well in folic acid and potassium.

3 cups shredded lettuce
1 cup shredded fresh spinach
1 small red or yellow sweet pepper, chopped
3 tablespoons sliced pitted ripe olives
1½ cups chopped cooked chicken
1 small tomato, chopped
Avocado Dressing

▲ In a large bowl toss together the lettuce, spinach, sweet pepper, and olives. Divide greens among 4 dinner plates. Top with chopped chicken and tomato. Serve with Avocado Dressing. Makes 4 servings.

Avocado Dressing: In a blender container or food processor bowl combine 1 small *ripe avocado*, seeded, peeled, and cut up; ¼ cup *plain nonfat yogurt*; 1 small fresh *jalapeño pepper*, stemmed and cut up; 1 *green onion*, cut up; 1 tablespoon snipped *cilantro or parsley*; 2 tablespoon *lemon or lime juice*; ⅓ cup *skim milk*; 1 clove *garlic*; and a dash *salt*. Cover and blend or process till smooth, scraping the sides of the container or bowl as necessary. Add additional *milk* if necessary, to make of drizzling consistency. Cover the surface with plastic wrap and chill up to 24 hours. Makes 1½ cups.

Nutrition Facts *per serving*: 206 calories, 10 g total fat (2 g saturated fat), 52 mg cholesterol, 154 mg sodium, 9 g carbohydrate, 3 g fiber, 20 g protein.
Daily Values: 31% vitamin A, 78% vitamin C, 8% calcium, 12% iron.

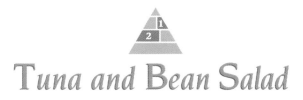

Tuna and Bean Salad

1 **8-ounce can cut green beans, rinsed and drained**
1 **8-ounce can cut wax beans, rinsed and drained**
½ **cup chopped green sweet pepper**
½ **cup sliced celery**
   Dijon Vinaigrette
1 **7-ounce can solid white tuna, drained**
4 **lettuce leaves (optional)**

▲ In a medium mixing bowl combine green and wax beans, green pepper, and celery. Pour Dijon Vinaigrette over bean mixture. Toss gently to coat. Gently fold in tuna. Cover and refrigerate 3 to 24 hours. If desired, serve on lettuce-lined plates. Makes 4 servings.

Dijon Vinaigrette: In a screw-top jar combine ¼ cup *water*; 3 tablespoons *lemon juice*; 4 teaspoons *Dijon-style mustard*; 1 tablespoon *olive or salad oil*; 1 teaspoon snipped *fresh thyme or* ¼ teaspoon *dried thyme*, crushed; and 1 clove *garlic*, minced. Cover and shake well to combine.

Nutrition Facts per serving: 139 calories, 5 g total fat (1 g saturated fat), 22 mg cholesterol, 520 mg sodium, 7 g carbohydrate, 2 g fiber, 16 g protein.
Daily Values: 6% vitamin A, 59% vitamin C, 3% calcium, 8% iron.

What a nice break from the usual sandwich. The tuna dresses up a bean salad for an extra special lunch. Tuna is a source of B$_{12}$, which is found only in foods from animals.

Tuna Tips

Canned tuna is available packed in oil or water. The oil-packed versions can contain as much as 13 grams of fat per 3-ounce serving. Water-packed tuna may have less than 1 gram fat per serving. If you're sodium-conscious, use lower-sodium, canned tuna in this recipe to slash the sodium by as much as 180 milligrams per serving.

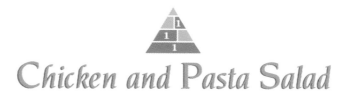

Chicken and Pasta Salad

This main-dish salad is a lunchtime treat—and it provides most of your vitamin C requirement for the day.

1 cup fresh or frozen sugar snap peas
6 ounces fine noodles or spaghetti
4 ounces asparagus spears, trimmed and cut into 1-inch pieces (about ½ cup)
⅓ cup bottled plum sauce
1 to 2 tablespoons light soy sauce
½ teaspoon toasted sesame oil
⅛ teaspoon crushed red pepper
1 cup chopped cooked chicken
1 medium red or green sweet pepper, cut into strips
1 11-ounce can mandarin orange sections, drained
⅓ cup sliced green onion
⅓ cup slivered almonds, toasted

▲ Thaw snap peas, if frozen. Halve peas crosswise. Set aside.

▲ Cook pasta according to package directions, except add the asparagus the last 4 to 6 minutes of cooking time. Drain.

▲ For dressing, in a small mixing bowl stir together plum sauce, soy sauce, sesame oil, and crushed red pepper. In a bowl combine cooked pasta and asparagus, peas, chicken, sweet pepper, oranges, onion, and almonds. Add dressing; toss to coat. Serve immediately. Makes 5 servings.

Nutrition Facts per serving: 297 calories, 8 g total fat (1 g saturated fat), 56 mg cholesterol, 150 mg sodium, 41 g carbohydrate, 2 g fiber, 16 g protein.
Daily Values: 21% vitamin A, 86% vitamin C, 4% calcium, 20% iron.

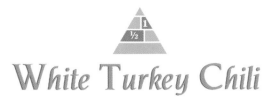

White Turkey Chili

1 cup frozen loose-pack whole kernel corn
1 large onion, chopped (1 cup)
3 cups water
2 cups chopped cooked turkey or chicken
1 15-ounce can great northern or cannellini beans, rinsed and drained
1 4-ounce can diced green chili peppers
2 teaspoons instant chicken bouillon granules
1 teaspoon ground cumin
  Several dashes bottled hot pepper sauce
  Shredded reduced-fat Monterey Jack cheese (optional)
  Snipped parsley (optional)

▲ In a large saucepan combine corn, onion, water, turkey or chicken, beans, chili peppers, bouillon granules, cumin, and hot pepper sauce. Bring to boiling; reduce heat. Simmer, covered, about 10 minutes or till vegetables are tender. To serve, ladle chili into serving bowls. If desired, top each serving with cheese and parsley. Makes 6 servings.

Nutrition Facts per serving: 187 calories, 6 g total fat (1 g saturated fat), 48 mg cholesterol, 492 mg sodium, 19 g carbohydrate, 4 g fiber, 20 g protein.
Daily Values: 4% vitamin A, 17% vitamin C, 5% calcium, 17% iron.

Thanks to the beans in this heart-healthy chili, one serving contains 16% of your fiber needs for the day, or about 4 grams of fiber per ½-cup serving.

Timesaving Poultry Pointers

For convenience, when a recipe calls for chopped cooked turkey or chicken, use canned (water-packed) chunk-style turkey or chicken,* drained; purchased deli-cooked chicken, boned and skinned; your own cut-up leftover cooked turkey or chicken; or purchased frozen chopped cooked chicken.
    *Note: One 5-ounce can of chunk-style chicken or turkey is equal to a generous ½ cup of chopped, cooked fresh chicken.

Quick-to-Fix Turkey and Rice Soup

A *great source of complex carbohydrates, rice is generally enriched with calcium, iron, and B vitamins.*

4 cups reduced-sodium chicken broth
1 cup water
1 teaspoon snipped fresh rosemary or ¼ teaspoon dried rosemary, crushed
¼ teaspoon pepper
1 10-ounce package frozen mixed vegetables (2 cups)
1 cup quick-cooking rice
2 cups chopped cooked turkey or chicken
1 16-ounce can tomatoes, cut up

▲ In a large saucepan or Dutch oven combine chicken broth, water, rosemary, and pepper. Bring to boiling.

▲ Stir in mixed vegetables and *uncooked* rice. Return to boiling. Reduce heat and simmer, covered, for 10 to 15 minutes or till vegetables and the rice are tender. Stir in turkey or chicken and *undrained* tomatoes. Heat through. To serve, ladle into serving bowls. Makes 6 servings.

Nutrition Facts per serving: 209 calories, 4 g total fat (1 g saturated fat), 36 mg cholesterol, 699 mg sodium, 24 g carbohydrate, 2 g fiber, 20 g protein.
Daily Values: 31% vitamin A, 23% vitamin C, 7% calcium, 18% iron.

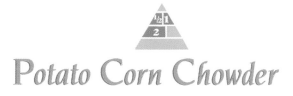

Potato Corn Chowder

2 cups loose-pack frozen whole kernel corn

2 cups loose-pack frozen diced hash brown potatoes with onions and peppers

1½ cups water

1 teaspoon instant chicken bouillon granules

⅛ to ¼ teaspoon white or black pepper

2 cloves garlic, minced

1 12-ounce can (1½ cups) evaporated skim milk

2 tablespoons all-purpose flour

½ cup finely chopped lower-sodium fully-cooked ham

Snipped parsley (optional)

▲ In a large saucepan combine corn, potatoes, water, bouillon granules, pepper, and garlic; bring to boiling. Reduce heat and cook, covered, about 5 minutes or till tender. *Do not drain.* Gradually stir the milk into the flour; add milk mixture to saucepan. Cook and stir till thickened and bubbly; cook and stir 1 minute more. Stir in the ham and heat through. To serve, ladle soup into serving bowls. If desired, sprinkle with snipped parsley. Makes 4 servings.

Nutrition Facts per serving: 256 calories, 6 g total fat (2 g saturated fat), 10 mg cholesterol, 529 mg sodium, 41 g carbohydrate, 2 g fiber, 14 g protein.
Daily Values: 16% vitamin A, 42% vitamin C, 22% calcium, 11% iron.

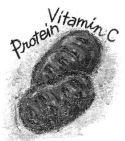

The humble potato isn't so humble nutritionally. If you skip the butter and sour cream, the potato is a nutrition gem, blessed with vitamins C and B$_6$, iron, and potassium. What's more, a small potato, with the skin left on, has about 2 grams of fiber.

What a Ham

The salty flavor of ham comes from the salt used to cure the meat. (If you're watching sodium intake, choose hams labeled "lower sodium.") After curing, most hams are smoked by suspending them in a smokehouse over hardwood fires that cook and give the meat a smoky flavor. Processing of most hams ends here, but a few are aged for several months to over a year. Most hams are labeled "fully cooked." This means they have been cooked during processing and are ready to eat with or without further heating.

Mexican Black Bean and Rice Soup

Complex carbohydrates (starches) abound in this meatless soup with beans and rice. Don't be afraid to eat starches—they're not fattening. They're rich in fiber and nutrition. At 11 grams of fiber, a serving of this soup supplies almost half of your fiber for the day.

2 **15-ounce cans black beans, rinsed and drained**
1 **14½-ounce can reduced-sodium chicken broth**
1 **medium onion, chopped (½ cup)**
½ **cup chopped red or green sweet pepper**
1 **tablespoon snipped cilantro (optional)**
¼ **teaspoon ground red pepper**
⅛ **teaspoon ground cumin**
2 **cloves garlic, minced**
2 **cups hot cooked rice**
½ **cup finely chopped, seeded tomato**
¼ **cup chopped avocado**

▲ In a large saucepan slightly mash the drained beans with a potato masher. Stir in chicken broth, onion, sweet pepper, cilantro (if desired), ground red pepper, cumin, and garlic.

▲ Bring the mixture to boiling. Reduce heat. Simmer, covered, for 10 minutes, stirring occasionally.

▲ To serve, divide cooked rice among 4 serving bowls. Ladle soup into bowls and top with tomato and avocado. Makes 4 servings.

Nutrition Facts per serving: 291 calories, 3 g total fat (0 g saturated fat), 0 mg cholesterol, 820 mg sodium, 58 g carbohydrate, 11 g fiber, 18 g protein.
Daily Values: 12% vitamin A, 48% vitamin C, 7% calcium, 24% iron.

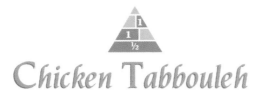

Chicken Tabbouleh

½ cup bulgur
1½ cups chopped cooked chicken or turkey
¾ cup coarsely chopped, seeded cucumber
½ cup sliced green onion
¼ cup snipped fresh parsley
3 tablespoons lemon juice
2 tablespoons water
1 tablespoon snipped fresh mint or 1 teaspoon dried mint, crushed
1 tablespoon olive oil or salad oil
⅛ teaspoon garlic salt
⅛ teaspoon pepper
1 large tomato, chopped

▲ Rinse bulgur in a colander with cold water; drain. In a medium mixing bowl combine bulgur, chicken or turkey, cucumber, green onions, and parsley. Set aside.

▲ For dressing, in a screw-top jar combine lemon juice, water, mint, oil, garlic salt, and pepper. Cover and shake well. Pour dressing over bulgur mixture. Toss lightly to coat. Cover and chill for 4 to 24 hours.

▲ Before serving, stir chopped tomato into bulgur mixture. Makes 4 servings.

Nutrition Facts per serving: 215 calories, 8 g total fat (2 g saturated fat), 51 mg cholesterol, 123 mg sodium, 17 g carbohydrate, 5 g fiber, 19 g protein.
Daily Values: 8% vitamin A, 37% vitamin C, 2% calcium, 12% iron.

Bulgur is a minimally processed wheat berry. High in nutrition and fiber, it gives this Middle Eastern main dish a nutty flavor.

Tabbouleh to Go

This recipe can be made ahead to tote to work or school for lunch. Just prepare it the night before, but do not add the tomato. Cover and chill the mixture overnight. In the morning, place the mixture in a cold insulated vacuum container and top the mixture with the chopped tomato. Before eating, stir in the tomatoes.

Ratatouille Ravioli

Eggplant, a colorful relative of the potato, offers high fiber content, especially when you cook it unpeeled.

1 **medium eggplant, cubed (about 3 cups)**
2 **small zucchini, halved lengthwise and cut into ¼-inch-thick slices (2 cups)**
1 **14½-ounce can low-sodium tomatoes, cut up**
1 **medium onion, chopped (½ cup)**
½ **cup chopped green sweet pepper**
1 **teaspoon dried basil, crushed**
½ **teaspoon dried thyme, crushed**
¼ **teaspoon garlic salt**
⅛ **teaspoon pepper**
1 **9-ounce package refrigerated cheese-filled ravioli**
2 **tablespoons grated Parmesan cheese**

▲ In a large saucepan combine the eggplant, zucchini, *undrained* tomatoes, onion, green pepper, basil, thyme, garlic salt, and pepper. Bring to boiling; reduce heat. Simmer, covered, about 20 minutes or till vegetables are tender. Cook, uncovered, for 5 to 10 minutes more or till of desired consistency, stirring occasionally.

▲ Meanwhile, cook ravioli according to package directions; drain. Add cooked ravioli to vegetable mixture; toss gently to combine. Sprinkle each serving with Parmesan cheese. Makes 4 servings.

Nutrition Facts per serving: 274 calories, 10 g total fat (5 g saturated fat), 59 mg cholesterol, 474 mg sodium, 36 g carbohydrate, 4 g fiber, 13 g protein.
Daily Values: 10% vitamin A, 48% vitamin C, 19% calcium, 15% iron.

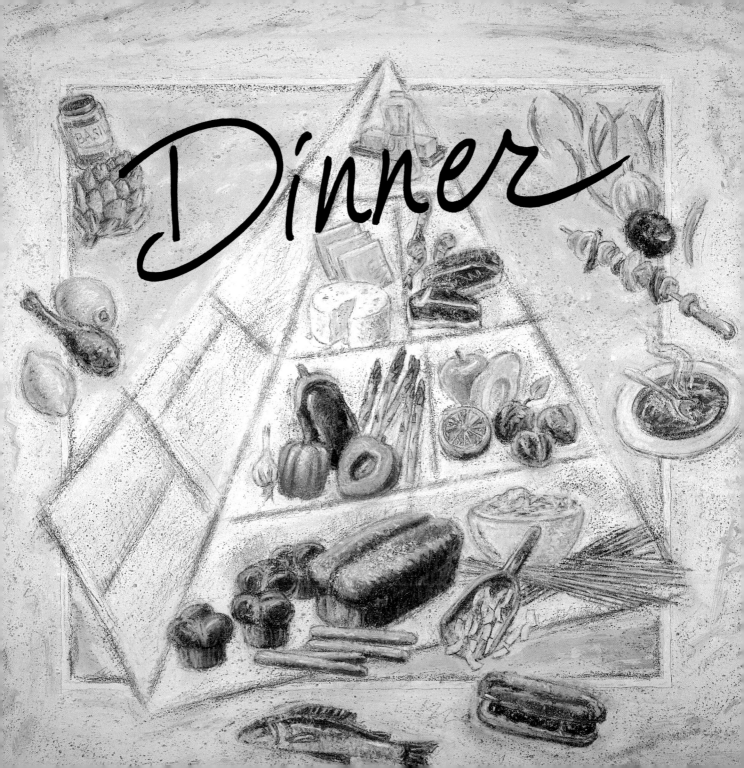

Dinner Menus

Monday
Tex-Mex Pot Roast
  (page 63)
Hot cooked rice
Steamed broccoli
Flour tortillas
Skim milk

Tuesday
Turkey Chimichangas (page 58)
Cheesy Beans (page 69)
Mixed greens salad
Cinnamon Fruit Compote
  (page 89)
Skim milk

Wednesday
Chinese-Style Turkey Burgers
  (page 53)
Potato Fries (page 88)
Plum-Sauced Sundaes (page 90)
Sparkling water

Thursday
Easy Shrimp Gumbo (page 73)
Hot cooked rice
Mixed greens salad
Chocolate Baked Pears (page 88)
Skim milk

Friday
Jerk Chicken with Chutney
  (page 45)
Rice Pilaf
Steamed carrots
Skim milk

Saturday
Pasta with Artichokes and Basil
  (page 79)
Mixed greens salad
Toasted baguette slices
Sparkling water

Sunday
Pork with Pear Sauce (page 64)
Wild rice
Snappy Green Beans (page 69)
Praline Baked Apples (page 91)
Sparkling water

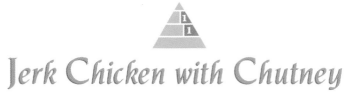

Jerk Chicken with Chutney

4 skinless, boneless chicken breast halves (about 1 pound total)
1 medium onion, chopped (½ cup)
3 tablespoons lime juice
1 tablespoon water
1 tablespoon Jamaican Jerk seasoning*
¼ teaspoon salt
⅓ cup chutney
1 large ripe banana, coarsely chopped
1 large ripe peach, peeled and chopped, or ¾ cup chopped frozen unsweetened peach slices, thawed

▲ Rinse the chicken; pat dry. In a blender container combine the onion, 2 *tablespoons* of the lime juice, the water, Jamaican Jerk seasoning, and salt. Cover and blend till pureed. Place chicken in a shallow dish. Add puree; turn to coat both sides of chicken. Cover and chill about 30 minutes.

▲ Meanwhile, in a small bowl combine the chutney, banana, peach and the remaining 1 tablespoon lime juice. Set aside. (You may cover the mixture and chill it for up to 2 hours.)

▲ Remove chicken from the puree, reserving puree. Place the chicken on the grill rack of an uncovered grill. Grill directly over *medium* coals for 12 to 15 minutes or till chicken is tender and no longer pink, turning and brushing once with puree. Serve chicken with chutney mixture. Makes 4 servings.

*Note: To make your own Jamaican Jerk seasoning, in a small bowl combine 1 teaspoon crushed *red pepper*, ½ teaspoon ground *allspice*, ¼ teaspoon *curry powder*, ¼ teaspoon *black pepper*, ⅛ teaspoon crushed dried *thyme*, and ⅛ teaspoon ground *red pepper*, and ⅛ teaspoon ground *ginger*.

Nutrition Facts per serving: 229 calories, 3 g total fat (1 g saturated fat), 59 mg cholesterol, 199 mg sodium, 27 g carbohydrate, 2 g fiber, 23 g protein.
Daily Values: 7% vitamin A, 17% vitamin C, 2% calcium, 8% iron.

Jamaican spices season the chicken, while the chutney enhances the flavors of this lively Caribbean dish. It adds up to a serving from both the Pyramid Meat and Fruit Groups.

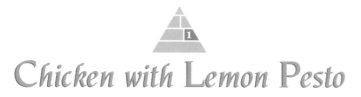

Chicken with Lemon Pesto

Made with less oil, this pesto is lower in fat but still loaded with flavor when compared to regular pesto.

Reduced-Fat Pesto
1 **tablespoon chicken broth or water**
¼ **teaspoon finely shredded lemon peel**
1 **teaspoon lemon juice**
  Nonstick spray coating
4 **medium skinless, boneless chicken breast halves (12 ounces total)**
  Pepper
  Pine nuts (optional)

▲ In a small bowl stir together ¼ *cup* of the Reduced-Fat Pesto, the chicken broth or water, lemon peel, and lemon. (Cover and chill remaining pesto for another use or use in Pesto Pasta Primavera, *page* 78.) Let stand at room temperature while preparing chicken.

▲ Spray a cold skillet with nonstick spray coating. Preheat skillet over medium heat. Sprinkle chicken lightly with pepper. Cook chicken in hot skillet for 10 to 13 minutes or till chicken is tender and no longer pink, turning once.

▲ To serve, transfer chicken to dinner plates. Spoon pesto mixture over chicken. If desired, sprinkle with a few pine nuts. Makes 4 servings.

Reduced-Fat Pesto: In a blender container or food processor bowl combine 1 cup firmly packed *fresh basil leaves*, ½ cup torn *fresh spinach leaves*, ¼ cup grated *Parmesan or Romano cheese*, ¼ cup *pine nuts or almonds*, 2 quartered cloves *garlic*, and ¼ teaspoon *salt*. Cover and blend or process with several on-off turns till a paste forms, stopping machine several times and scraping sides as necessary. With machine running, gradually add 2 tablespoons *olive oil or cooking oil* and 2 tablespoons *water*; blend or process till mixture is the consistency of soft butter. Transfer to a storage container. Cover and refrigerate up to 2 days or divide into ¼-cup portions and freeze up to 1 month. Makes ¾ cup.

Nutrition Facts per serving: 170 calories, 8 g total fat (2 g saturated fat), 61 mg cholesterol, 151 mg sodium, 1 g carbohydrate, 0 g fiber, 24 g protein.
Daily Values: 2% vitamin A, 2% vitamin C, 4% calcium, 7% iron.

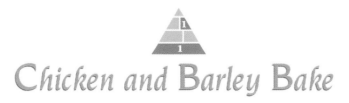

Chicken and Barley Bake

1 large onion, chopped (1 cup)
¾ cup chopped carrot
¾ cup water
½ cup pearl barley
1½ teaspoons instant chicken bouillon granules
½ teaspoon poultry seasoning
1 clove garlic, minced
1½ pounds chicken thighs, skinned
2 tablespoons snipped parsley or sage

▲ In a medium saucepan combine onion, carrot, water, barley, bouillon granules, poultry seasoning, and garlic. Heat mixture to boiling.

▲ Pour hot mixture into a 1½-quart casserole. Arrange chicken thighs atop mixture.

▲ Bake, covered, in a 350° oven for 1 hour or till barley is tender and chicken is no longer pink. Sprinkle with parsley. Makes 4 servings.

Nutrition Facts per serving: 221 calories, 6 g total fat (2 g saturated fat), 49 mg cholesterol, 400 mg sodium, 24 g carbohydrate, 5 g fiber, 17 g protein.
Daily Values: 90% vitamin A, 7% vitamin C, 3% calcium, 13% iron.

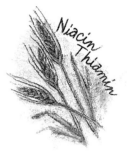

One serving of this easy dish gives you 5 grams of fiber, which is about 20% of your 25-gram goal for the entire day.

Oh, Barley

Barley, a cereal grain with a stellar past, has been around for centuries. In fact, it was cultivated in Egypt between 6000 and 5000 B.C. and was found in the tomb of the great Egyptian King Tut. The grain was used as currency, offered to the Egyptian gods as gifts, and made into necklaces for placing on mummies to symbolize resurrection. But barley deserves a place on your plate, too. It has been shown to contain an unidentified attribute that inhibits the production of cholesterol. Aside from that, barley contain niacin, thiamin, and potassium.

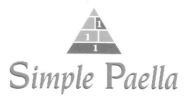

Simple Paella

Traditional paella gets its signature color from saffron, but we've substituted the more readily available turmeric to produce the same result. Artichoke hearts bestow fiber, calcium, and phosphorus to this dish.

1　6-ounce package frozen, peeled, cooked shrimp
2　cups water
1　cup long grain rice
1　medium onion, chopped (½ cup)
1½　teaspoons instant chicken bouillon granules
⅛　teaspoon ground turmeric
⅛　teaspoon ground red pepper
1　cup chopped cooked chicken
1　14-ounce can artichoke hearts, drained and halved
½　cup frozen loose-pack peas
2　tablespoons diced pimiento

▲ Thaw shrimp; set aside. In a large skillet combine water, *uncooked* rice, onion, bouillon granules, turmeric, and red pepper. Bring to boiling; reduce heat. Simmer, covered, for 15 minutes.

▲ Stir the thawed shrimp, chicken, artichoke hearts, peas, and pimiento into rice mixture. Cover and cook for 1 to 2 minutes more or till heated through. Makes 5 servings.

Nutrition Facts per serving: 272 calories, 3 g total fat (1 g saturated fat), 93 mg cholesterol, 453 mg sodium, 39 g carbohydrate, 4 g fiber, 21 g protein.
Daily Values: 5% vitamin A, 20% vitamin C, 5% calcium, 26% iron.

Seafood Savvy

Although fish and seafood contain cholesterol and saturated fat, it's generally a lot less than meat or even poultry. Fish can, and should, be enjoyed in a healthful diet. Fish and shellfish contain a type of unsaturated fat, called omega-3 fatty acids, which has been shown to be kind to your heart. But be sure to eat the real thing. Fish oil pills are high in fat and calories, and their long-term effects are unknown.

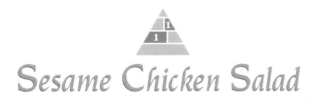

Sesame Chicken Salad

1 2- to 2½-pound whole
    deli-roasted chicken
1 10-ounce package torn mixed
    European-style or Italian-blend
    salad greens
1 8¾-ounce can whole baby corn,
    drained and cut in half
    crosswise
2 green onions, sliced (¼ cup)
¼ cup sliced radishes
½ cup orange juice
¼ cup rice vinegar or white vinegar
½ teaspoon toasted sesame oil
¼ teaspoon pepper
1½ teaspoons sesame seed, toasted

▲ Cut chicken into pieces. Remove skin and bones; discard. Shred enough chicken with 2 forks to make 2 cups. (Save the remaining chicken for another use.)

▲ In a large salad bowl combine the 2 cups shredded chicken, salad greens, baby corn, green onions, and radishes.

▲ For dressing, in a screw-top jar combine orange juice, rice vinegar, sesame oil, and pepper. Cover and shake well. Pour dressing over salad mixture, tossing lightly to coat. Sprinkle with sesame seed. Makes 6 servings.

Nutrition Facts per serving: 154 calories, 7 g total fat (2 g saturated fat), 53 mg cholesterol, 96 mg sodium, 6 g carbohydrate, 2 g fiber, 15 g protein.
Daily Values: 13% vitamin A, 26% vitamin C, 2% calcium, 8% iron.

Salad dressing doesn't have to be loaded with oil. The one used here has only a half teaspoon of sesame oil. It is strong in flavor, so a little goes a long way. Orange juice makes up the bulk of the dressing, adding vitamin C and folic acid.

Grilled Honey-Chicken Sandwiches

Vitamin B$_{12}$ plays an important role in the formation of red blood cells. It is only found in dairy products, eggs, fish, meat, and poultry, so be sure to eat the full number of servings from the Pyramid's Meat and Dairy Groups each day.

3 tablespoons orange juice
1 tablespoon light soy sauce
1 tablespoon honey
1 teaspoon lemon-pepper seasoning
½ teaspoon ground ginger
⅛ teaspoon garlic powder
2 large skinless, boneless chicken breast halves (8 ounces total)
2 whole wheat hamburger buns
   Lettuce leaves
   Pineapple slices (optional)

▲ In a shallow dish combine the orange juice, soy sauce, honey, lemon-pepper seasoning, ginger, and garlic powder. Set aside.

▲ Place chicken breasts between 2 sheets of plastic wrap. Pound each with a meat mallet until ½ inch thick; place in marinade. Cover; refrigerate for 4 to 6 hours or overnight, turning bag occasionally.

▲ At serving time, remove chicken from marinade, discarding marinade. Place chicken on an uncovered grill directly over *medium-hot* coals. Grill about 10 minutes or till the chicken is tender and no longer pink, turning halfway through cooking time. (Or, place chicken on the unheated rack of a broiler pan. Broil 4 to 5 inches from heat for 6 to 7 minutes, turning halfway through cooking.)

▲ Split buns and place on grill rack or broiler pan for 1 to 2 minutes to toast. Serve chicken breasts on toasted buns. Top each serving with lettuce and, if desired, pineapple slices. Makes 2 servings.

Nutrition Facts per serving: 277 calories, 6 g total fat (2 g saturated fat), 59 mg cholesterol, 703 mg sodium, 29 g carbohydrate, 1 g fiber, 27 g protein.
Daily Values: 3% vitamin A, 23% vitamin C, 5% calcium, 19% iron.

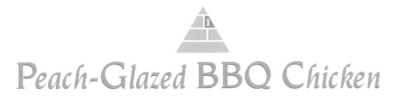

Peach-Glazed BBQ Chicken

2 to 2½ pounds meaty chicken pieces (breasts, thighs, and drumsticks)
½ cup peach spreadable fruit
3 tablespoons vinegar
2 teaspoons Worcestershire sauce
¼ teaspoon ground cinnamon
⅛ teaspoon ground allspice

▲ Skin chicken pieces. Rinse chicken; pat dry with paper towels. Arrange *medium-hot* coals around drip pan; test for *medium* heat above drip pan. Place chicken, bone side up, on the grill rack over drip pan. Cover grill and cook the chicken for 50 to 60 minutes or till chicken is tender and no longer pink, brushing the chicken occasionally with the glaze during the last 10 minutes of grilling.

▲ For glaze, in a small saucepan combine the spreadable fruit, vinegar, Worcestershire sauce, cinnamon, and allspice. Heat and stir just till the spreadable fruit melts.

▲ To serve, spoon any remaining glaze over chicken. Makes 4 servings.

Nutrition Facts per serving: 304 calories, 7 g total fat (2 g saturated fat), 92 mg cholesterol, 112 mg sodium, 29 g carbohydrate, 0 g fiber, 30 g protein.
Daily Values: 1% vitamin A, 7% vitamin C, 2% calcium, 12% iron.

This barbecued chicken is just peachy—helping you work toward your Pyramid Meat Group servings for the day. Try other fruit flavors for variety. Look for fruit spreads that contain all fruit.

Grilled Fruit

To up your fruit ante, grill some fresh peach halves or pineapple slices alongside the chicken during the last 7 to 10 minutes of cooking time.

Turkey-Stuffed Acorn Squash

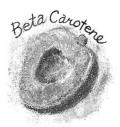
Beta Carotene

In general, dark yellow and green fruits and vegetables, such as acorn squash, boast high beta carotene content. The deeper the color, the more they contain. Beta carotene is believed to help decrease risk of heart disease and cancer and slow the process of aging.

2 medium acorn squash (about 1 pound each)

12 ounces ground raw turkey

⅓ cup chopped onion

¼ teaspoon garlic salt

¼ teaspoon dried Italian seasoning, crushed

⅛ teaspoon pepper

½ of an 8-ounce package (4 ounces) fat-free cream cheese, cut up

2 tablespoons skim milk

2 tablespoons fine dry bread crumbs

1 teaspoon margarine or butter, melted

▲ Halve squash lengthwise. Remove seeds. Place squash, cut side down, in a shallow baking dish. Bake in a 350° oven for 30 minutes.

▲ Meanwhile, in a large skillet cook turkey, onion, garlic salt, Italian seasoning, and pepper till no pink remains. Drain off fat. Stir in cream cheese till melted. Add milk.

▲ Turn squash cut side up. Spoon turkey mixture into squash halves. Stir together the bread crumbs and melted margarine; sprinkle over turkey filling. Bake, uncovered, for 20 to 25 minutes more or till squash is tender. Makes 4 servings.

Nutrition Facts per serving: 228 calories, 8 g total fat (2 g saturated fat), 36 mg cholesterol, 212 mg sodium, 24 g carbohydrate, 4 g fiber, 18 g protein.
Daily Values: 128% vitamin A, 43% vitamin C, 16% calcium, 14% iron.

Top Turkey Tips

Store-bought ground turkey or chicken often contains poultry skin, which has a high fat content. When buying ground poultry, choose a brand without the skin. If it's not available, ask your butcher to grind fresh turkey or chicken for you, or grind your own at home.

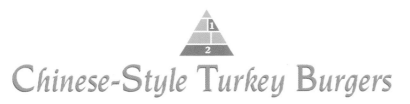

Chinese-Style Turkey Burgers

1   **beaten egg**
½   **cup fine dry bread crumbs**
¼   **cup finely chopped peanuts or water chestnuts**
1   **tablespoon light soy sauce**
¼   **teaspoon ground ginger**
⅛   **teaspoon pepper**
1   **pound ground raw turkey or chicken**
⅓   **cup orange marmalade spreadable fruit**
1½ **teaspoons light soy sauce or teriyaki sauce**
4   **whole wheat hamburger buns, split and toasted**
4   **lettuce leaves or Chinese cabbage leaves**

▲ In a medium mixing bowl combine egg, bread crumbs, peanuts or water chestnuts, the 1 tablespoon soy sauce, ginger, and pepper. Add ground turkey or chicken; mix well. Shape into six ½-inch-thick patties.

▲ Grill patties on the grill rack of an uncovered grill directly over *medium* coals for 11 to 13 minutes or till juices run clear, turning once halfway through grilling time.

▲ Meanwhile, for sauce, in a small saucepan stir together the orange marmalade and 1½ teaspoons soy or teriyaki sauce. Cook and stir over low heat just till marmalade melts.

▲ Just before serving, brush sauce onto burgers. Serve on buns; top with lettuce or cabbage leaves. Makes 6 servings.

Nutrition Facts per serving: 280 calories, 9 g total fat (2 g saturated fat), 64 mg cholesterol, 377 mg sodium, 34 g carbohydrate, 2 g fiber, 17 g protein.
Daily Values: 2% vitamin A, 2% vitamin C, 4% calcium, 14% iron.

Peanuts add flavor, crunch, and protein to these orange-glazed burgers. Although peanuts are a source of fat, the fat they contain is unsaturated, which is kinder to your heart and arteries.

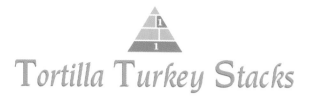

Tortilla Turkey Stacks

Although refried beans contain fat, the vegetarian version is made with vegetable oil rather than lard The high fiber and protein content of beans makes them an excellent meat substitute.

4   7-inch flour tortillas
1½ cups chopped cooked turkey or chicken
2   tablespoons nonfat Thousand Island salad dressing
2   tablespoons chunky-style salsa
1   tablespoon thinly sliced green onion
½   of a 16-ounce can vegetarian refried beans (about 1 cup)
3   cups shredded lettuce
1   medium tomato, chopped
¼   cup shredded reduced-fat Monterey Jack cheese (1 ounce)

▲ Place tortillas in a single layer on a baking sheet. Bake in a 350° oven for 10 to 12 minutes or till crisp and lightly browned. (If tortillas puff during baking, poke with a fork to allow steam to escape).

▲ Meanwhile, in a medium mixing bowl combine turkey or chicken, salad dressing, salsa, and green onion. Set aside.

▲ Spread about ¼ *cup* of the refried beans over *each* tortilla. Top with turkey mixture, shredded lettuce, and chopped tomato. Sprinkle each serving with shredded cheese. Makes 4 servings.

Nutrition Facts per serving: 321 calories, 9 g total fat (3 g saturated fat), 60 mg cholesterol, 603 mg sodium, 35 g carbohydrate, 3 g fiber, 26 g protein.
Daily Values: 6% vitamin A, 22% vitamin C, 11% calcium, 22% iron.

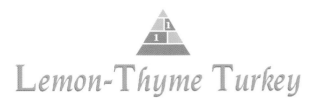

Lemon-Thyme Turkey

6 ounces turkey breast slices
¼ teaspoon finely shredded
    lemon peel
1 tablespoon lemon juice
2 teaspoons cooking oil
½ teaspoon instant chicken
    bouillon granules
⅛ teaspoon dried thyme, crushed
1 clove garlic, minced
    Dash salt
    Dash pepper
    Nonstick spray coating
1½ cups sliced zucchini and/or
    yellow summer squash
½ cup sliced fresh mushrooms
1½ teaspoons cornstarch
    Hot cooked rice (optional)

▲ If necessary, cut turkey into 2 equal portions.

▲ For marinade, in a small bowl stir together lemon peel, lemon juice, oil, bouillon granules, thyme, garlic, salt, pepper, and ¼ cup *water*.

▲ Place turkey in a plastic bag set in a bowl. Pour marinade over turkey. Close bag and refrigerate for 2 hours, turning bag occasionally.

▲ Remove the turkey from the bag, reserving marinade. Spray an 8-inch skillet with nonstick spray coating. Add turkey slices. Cook over medium heat about 4 minutes or till tender and no longer pink, turning once. Remove turkey from skillet; cover to keep warm.

▲ Add the zucchini, mushrooms, and 2 tablespoons *water* to the skillet. Cover and cook for 3 to 4 minutes or till zucchini is crisp-tender.

▲ Meanwhile, stir together the reserved marinade and cornstarch. Add to the vegetables in the skillet. Cook and stir till thickened and bubbly. Cook and stir 1 minute more. Serve the vegetables with turkey slices and, if desired, rice. Serves 2.

Nutrition Facts per serving: 161 calories, 7 g total fat (1 g saturated fat), 37 mg cholesterol, 321 mg sodium, 8 g carbohydrate, 2 g fiber, 17 g protein.
Daily Values: 2% vitamin A, 15% vitamin C, 2% calcium, 9% iron.

If served with a half cup of rice, this healthful main dish fulfills one serving each from the Pyramid's Bread, Meat, and Vegetable Groups.

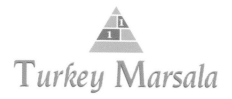

Turkey Marsala

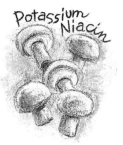
Potassium
Niacin

A cup of sliced mushrooms has just 18 calories and offers a healthy dose of potassium. Their earthy flavor lends a tempting taste to this simple, yet elegant entrée.

2 turkey breast tenderloins (about 1 pound)
1 tablespoon margarine or butter
2 cups sliced fresh mushrooms
½ cup reduced-sodium chicken broth
¼ cup dry marsala or apple juice
2 tablespoons snipped parsley

▲ Cut the tenderloins horizontally to make 4 portions. If desired, sprinkle steaks with salt and pepper.

▲ In a large skillet melt the margarine or butter. Cook turkey over medium heat for 7 to 9 minutes or till tender and no longer pink, turning halfway through cooking. Remove turkey from skillet; keep warm.

▲ Cook mushrooms in skillet drippings till tender. Carefully stir in broth and marsala or apple juice. Bring to boiling. Boil rapidly for 3 to 4 minutes (you should have about ¾ cup mixture). Stir in parsley. To serve, spoon mushroom mixture over turkey steaks. Makes 4 servings.

Nutrition Facts per serving: 171 calories, 5 g total fat (1 g saturated fat), 50 mg cholesterol, 161 mg sodium, 3 g carbohydrate, 0 g fiber, 23 g protein.
Daily Values: 4% vitamin A, 6% vitamin C, 1% calcium, 11% iron.

Mushroom Tip

Wipe mushrooms clean with a damp cloth or paper towel rather than rinsing them with water. Mushrooms are like little sponges; they'll soak up the water and water out when cooked, leaving you with a watery tasting dish.

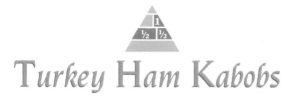

Turkey Ham Kabobs

12 pearl onions, peeled
 2 large green or red sweet
      peppers, cut into 1½-inch
      pieces
 1 pound full cooked turkey ham,
      cut into 1-inch chunks
 1 8¼-ounce can pineapple chunks
      (juice-packed), drained
 ½ cup low-calorie apricot spread
 1 tablespoon orange juice
 1 tablespoon prepared mustard
1½ teaspoons prepared horseradish

▲ In a small saucepan cook pearl onions, covered, in a small amount of boiling water for 2 minutes. Add green or red sweet peppers; cook for 1 minute more. Drain vegetables.

▲ On 6 long metal skewers alternately thread cooked onions and peppers, turkey ham, and pineapple chunks. Set aside.

▲ For glaze, in a small saucepan combine apricot spread, orange juice, mustard, and horseradish. Cook and stir over low heat till the apricot spread melts.

▲ Place kabobs on the unheated rack of a broiler pan. Broil 4 to 6 inches from heat for 8 to 12 minutes or till turkey ham is heated through, turning once and brushing 3 to 4 times with glaze. Makes 6 servings.

Nutrition Facts per serving: 207 calories, 4 g total fat (1 g saturated fat), 42 mg cholesterol, 806 mg sodium, 28 g carbohydrate, 2 g fiber, 15 g protein.
Daily Values: 10% vitamin A, 62% vitamin C, 2% calcium, 19% iron.

To meet the recommended two to four daily servings from the Pyramid Fruit Group, pair meats with fruit. In this family favorite, pineapple provides potassium, which has been shown to help control high blood pressure.

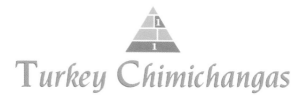

Turkey Chimichangas

Your family will surely rave about this baked version of a typically high-fat Mexican specialty. Added bonus: One tortilla makes up one serving from the Bread Group of the Pyramid, bringing you closer to your minimum of six servings a day.

1 teaspoon chili powder
¾ teaspoon ground cumin
¼ teaspoon salt
2 turkey breast tenderloins (about 1 pound total)
¾ cup shredded reduced-fat cheddar cheese (3 ounces)
½ cup fat-free dairy sour cream salsa dip
1 tablespoon snipped fresh cilantro (optional)
4 10-inch flour tortillas Nonstick spray coating
⅓ cup salsa Snipped cilantro (optional)

▲ In a small mixing bowl combine chili powder, cumin, and salt. Rinse turkey; pat dry. Halve the tenderloins horizontally to make 4 portions. Rub the cumin mixture onto both sides of turkey. Place the turkey on an unheated rack of a broiler pan. Broil 4 to 5 inches from heat for 5 minutes. Turn and broil 4 to 6 minutes more or till turkey is tender and no longer pink. Cut cooked turkey into thin strips. Set aside.

▲ In a medium mixing bowl combine the cheddar cheese, sour cream dip, and, if desired, cilantro. Stir turkey strips into cheese mixture. Set aside.

▲ For tortillas, wrap 2 tortillas at a time in microwave-safe paper towels. Microwave on 100% power (high) for 10 to 15 seconds. Repeat with the remaining 2 tortillas. (Or, wrap tortillas in foil and bake in a 350° oven for 15 minutes.)

▲ Spoon *one-fourth* of the turkey mixture onto *each* tortilla, near one edge. Fold edge nearest filling over the filling just till mixture is covered. Fold in the sides; roll up. Secure with toothpicks. Spray both sides of chimichangas with nonstick spray coating. Place chimichangas on a large baking sheet. Bake in a 450° oven for 7 to 10 minutes or till tortillas are crisp. To serve, top with salsa and, if desired, additional snipped cilantro. Makes 4 servings.

Nutrition Facts per serving: 328 calories, 8 g total fat (3 g saturated fat), 65 mg cholesterol, 618 mg sodium, 26 g carbohydrate, 0 g fiber, 32 g protein.
Daily Values: 12% vitamin A, 14% vitamin C, 21% calcium, 19% iron.

Grilled Steak and Kabobs

1   12-ounce bottle (1½ cups)
        nonalcoholic beer or
        regular beer
2   tablespoons light soy sauce
1   teaspoon ground cumin
1   to 2 teaspoons chili powder
2   cloves garlic, minced
1   pound boneless beef sirloin or
        top loin steak, cut
        1 inch thick
2   fresh ears of corn, husks
        removed and cut crosswise
        into 1-inch pieces
1   medium red onion, cut into
        wedges
2   medium zucchini, cut crosswise
        into ½-inch slices
1   red, yellow, or green sweet
        pepper, cut into 1-inch pieces

▲ For marinade, combine beer, soy sauce, cumin, chili powder, and garlic. Set aside.

▲ Trim fat from meat. Place steak in a plastic bag set in a shallow dish. Pour marinade over steak. Close bag. Marinate in refrigerator for 6 to 24 hours, turning bag occasionally.

▲ In a large saucepan cook corn in a small amount of boiling water, covered, for 3 minutes. Add onion wedges; cook, covered, 4 minutes more. Add zucchini and cook, covered, 1 minute more. Drain; cool slightly. Thread partially cooked vegetables and sweet pepper on four long skewers; set aside.

▲ Drain steak, reserving marinade. Grill steak and kabobs on the grill rack of an uncovered grill directly over *medium* coals to desired doneness, turning once and brushing with reserved marinade halfway through cooking time. (Allow 10 to 12 minutes for *medium-rare* and 12 to 15 minutes for *medium* doneness for meat; allow 10 to 12 minutes for vegetables.) To serve, cut steak into serving-size pieces. Serve with vegetable kabobs. Makes 4 servings.

Nutrition Facts per serving: 277 calories, 11 g total fat (4 g saturated fat), 76 mg cholesterol, 157 mg sodium, 16 g carbohydrate, 3 g fiber, 28 g protein.
Daily Values: 16% vitamin A, 62% vitamin C, 2% calcium, 24% iron.

Nonalcoholic beer lends a delicious flavor to this marinated steak dinner. Keep it lean by selecting sirloin or top loin steaks, which have about 7 to 8 grams of fat per 3-ounce serving.

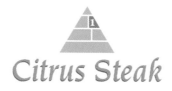

Citrus Steak

Lemon juice adds vitamin C and a burst of flavor to simple flank steak. Eating a vitamin C-rich food along with foods rich in iron, such as red meat, helps your body absorb the iron more readily. This, of course, is important to women of child-bearing age.

1   1½-pound flank steak or boneless beef top sirloin steak
1   teaspoon finely shredded lemon peel
½   cup lemon juice
2   tablespoons sugar
2   tablespoons light soy sauce
1½ teaspoons snipped fresh oregano or ½ teaspoon dried oregano, crushed
⅛   teaspoon pepper
    Grilled vegetables (optional, see box below)

▲ Score meat by making shallow cuts at 1-inch intervals diagonally across the steak in a diamond pattern; repeat on other side of meat. Place meat in a plastic bag set in a shallow bowl.

▲ For marinade, in a 1-cup glass measure stir together lemon peel, lemon juice, sugar, soy sauce, oregano, and pepper. Pour marinade over meat; close bag. Marinate in refrigerator for 2 hours or overnight.

▲ Drain meat, reserving marinade. Grill steak on an uncovered grill directly over *medium* coals for 12 to 14 minutes for *medium* doneness, turning once during cooking and brushing occasionally with marinade. Discard any remaining marinade. To serve, thinly slice meat diagonally across the grain. Makes 6 servings.

Nutrition Facts per serving: 182 calories, 8 g total fat (3 g saturated fat), 53 mg cholesterol, 295 mg sodium, 4 g carbohydrate, 0 g fiber, 22 g protein.
Daily Values: 0% vitamin A, 11% vitamin C, 0% calcium, 14% iron.

Grilled Vegetables

Cut fresh vegetables, such as zucchini, eggplant, or sweet peppers, into 1-inch pieces. Spray with nonstick spray coating. Place vegetables on a piece of heavy foil. Cover; grill zucchini for 5 to 6 minutes, eggplant about 8 minutes, and sweet peppers for 8 to 10 minutes, turning occasionally.

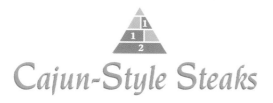

Cajun-Style Steaks

2 tablespoons all-purpose flour
½ to 1 teaspoon Cajun or blackened steak seasoning*
4 beef cubed steaks (about 1 pound total)
2 teaspoons cooking oil
1 14½-ounce can tomatoes, cut up
1 8-ounce can low-sodium tomato sauce
1½ teaspoons dried oregano, crushed
⅛ teaspoon salt
1 medium green pepper, cut into strips
1 small onion, sliced and separated into rings
2 cups hot cooked rice

▲ In a shallow dish combine the flour and Cajun or blackened steak seasoning. Dip steaks into flour mixture, coating both sides. In a large skillet brown meat in hot oil. (If all 4 steaks will not fit in the skillet, brown *half* at a time, adding an additional teaspoon of oil if needed for the second batch; return all meat to the skillet.)

▲ Add *undrained* tomatoes, tomato sauce, oregano, and salt to the skillet. Bring to boiling. Reduce heat and simmer, covered, for 25 minutes, stirring occasionally. Add green pepper and onion. Cover and simmer for 5 to 7 minutes more or till the meat and vegetables are tender. Skim fat from juices. Serve with hot cooked rice. Makes 4 servings.

*Note: To make your own blackened seasoning blend, in small bowl combine ½ teaspoon *onion powder*; ½ teaspoon *garlic powder*; ½ teaspoon ground *white pepper*; ½ teaspoon ground *red pepper*; ½ teaspoon ground *black pepper*; ½ teaspoon dried *thyme*, crushed; and ⅛ teaspoon *salt*. Store tightly covered in a cool place.

Nutrition Facts per serving: 357 calories, 8 g total fat (2 g saturated fat), 72 mg cholesterol, 327 mg sodium, 37 g carbohydrate, 2 g fiber, 32 g protein.
Daily Values: 14% vitamin A, 62% vitamin C, 5% calcium, 33% iron.

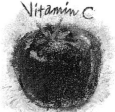

Vitamin C

This saucy dish includes both canned whole tomatoes and tomato sauce for a double dose of vitamin C.

Flank Steak with Horseradish Sauce

1   1- to 1½-pound beef flank steak
    or beef top round steak
⅓   cup nonfat Italian salad dressing
    Horseradish Sauce

▲ Score meat by making shallow cuts at 1-inch intervals diagonally across steak in a diamond pattern. Repeat on other side of meat. Place meat in a plastic bag set in a shallow bowl. Pour salad dressing over meat. Close bag. Marinate steak in refrigerator for 4 to 24 hours, turning occasionally.

▲ Drain meat, discarding marinade. Place meat on the unheated rack of a broiler pan. Broil 3 inches from heat to desired doneness, turning once halfway through cooking time. (Allow 15 to 16 minutes for *medium*.)

▲ To serve, thinly slice meat diagonally across the grain. Serve with Horseradish Sauce. Store any remaining sauce in an airtight container for up to 5 days. Makes 4 to 6 servings.

Horseradish Sauce: In a small saucepan combine ½ cup *fat-free dairy sour cream*, ½ cup *nonfat mayonnaise dressing or salad dressing*, 1 tablespoon *nonfat Italian salad dressing*, 1 tablespoon *prepared horseradish*, 1 tablespoon snipped *parsley*, 1 tablespoon *skim milk*, and ¼ teaspoon *pepper*. Cook and stir over low heat just till heated through. *Do not boil.*

Nutrition Facts per serving with 2 tablespoons Horseradish Sauce: 203 calories, 8 g total fat (3 g saturated fat), 53 mg cholesterol, 594 mg sodium, 7 g carbohydrate, 0 g fiber, 23 g protein.
Daily Values: 2% vitamin A, 1% vitamin C, 2% calcium, 14% iron.

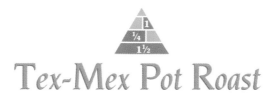

Tex-Mex Pot Roast

Nonstick spray coating
1 2- to 2½-pound beef bottom
     round roast
1 14½-ounce can Mexican-style
     stewed tomatoes
1 medium onion, chopped (½ cup)
1 tablespoon chili powder
¼ teaspoon salt
¼ teaspoon pepper
¼ teaspoon ground cinnamon
2 cloves garlic, minced
3 cups hot cooked rice or noodles

▲ Spray a 4- to 4½-quart Dutch oven with nonstick coating. Preheat over medium heat. Place meat in pan; brown meat on all sides. Drain off fat.

▲ Stir together the *undrained* tomatoes, onion, chili powder, salt, pepper, cinnamon, and garlic; pour over meat in Dutch oven. Bake, covered, in a 325° oven for 1½ to 2 hours or till meat is tender.

▲ To serve, slice meat. Serve meat with hot cooked rice or noodles. Spoon tomato mixture over meat and rice. Makes 8 to 10 servings.

Nutrition Facts per serving: 280 calories, 8 g total fat (3 g saturated fat), 77 mg cholesterol, 294 mg sodium, 22 g carbohydrate, 1 g fiber, 28 g protein.
Daily Values: 7% vitamin A, 15% vitamin C, 2% calcium, 26% iron.

To choose the leanest beef, look for cuts from the loin (such as tenderloin or strip loin) or round (such as top or bottom round or eye of round). Trim all visible fat before cooking.

How Lean It Is

Red meat can be part of a low-fat diet as long as you choose lean cuts. Thanks to new breeding and feeding techniques, such cuts are more readily available today. Butchers are doing their part, too, by trimming fat more closely. As a result, calories, fat, and cholesterol have all been slashed. Choose the following for the leanest cuts:

Bottom round roast   Round tip roast
Top round steak or roast   T-bone steak
Eye round roast   Top loin steak
Arm pot roast   Sirloin steak

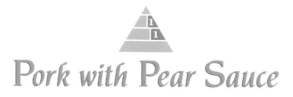

Pork with Pear Sauce

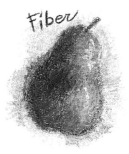

A touch of nutmeg makes this pear sauce a sweet complement to pork. Leave the skin on the pears for maximum fiber content.

2 medium pears, cored and sliced
  Pear nectar or orange juice
    (about 1 cup)
1 tablespoon cooking oil
4 boneless pork loin chops, cut
    1 inch thick (12 ounces total)
1 tablespoon all-purpose flour
1 tablespoon Dijon-style mustard
1 teaspoon coarsely ground whole
    black pepper
¼ teaspoon ground nutmeg
  Coarsely ground whole black
    pepper

▲ In a medium saucepan cook pear slices, covered, in pear nectar or orange juice for 5 to 7 minutes or till tender. Remove with a slotted spoon, reserving liquid. Cover pears; keep warm. Measure liquid; if necessary, add pear nectar or orange juice to equal 1 cup. Set aside.

▲ In a 10-inch skillet heat cooking oil over medium-high heat. Add pork chops; reduce heat to medium. Cook, uncovered, for 10 to 12 minutes or till the center is just slightly pink, turning once during cooking. Remove the chops from skillet, reserving drippings in skillet.

▲ Stir flour into reserved drippings. Stir in reserved nectar, the mustard, the 1 teaspoon black pepper, and the nutmeg. Cook and stir till thickened and bubbly. Cook and stir for 1 minute more. To serve, place chops on dinner plates; arrange pears around chops. Spoon sauce over chops; sprinkle with additional black pepper. Makes 4 servings.

Nutrition Facts per serving: 230 calories, 10 g total fat (2 g saturated fat), 38 mg cholesterol, 126 mg sodium, 24 g carbohydrate, 2 g fiber, 13 g protein.
Daily Values: 0% vitamin A, 7% vitamin C, 1% calcium, 6% iron.

Pork Kabobs with Yogurt Sauce

1 16-ounce container plain nonfat
    yogurt
2 tablespoons lemon juice
2 to 4 cloves garlic, minced
1 tablespoon snipped fresh
    oregano or 2 teaspoons dried
    oregano, crushed
1 tablespoon snipped fresh mint or
    1 teaspoon dried mint, crushed
1½ pounds boneless pork loin, cut
    into 1-inch cubes
½ cup finely chopped, seeded
    tomato
½ cup seeded, finely chopped
    cucumber
4 cups fresh vegetables (such as
    eggplant, zucchini, yellow
    summer squash, red onion,
    and mushrooms), cut into
    1-inch pieces
    Olive-oil-flavored or regular
    nonstick spray coating

▲ In a medium bowl combine yogurt, lemon juice, garlic, 1 *teaspoon* of the oregano, and mint. Divide mixture in half. Stir the pork cubes into *half* of the yogurt mixture. Cover and chill meat and remaining yogurt mixture for 1 to 4 hours.

▲ For sauce, up to 1 hour before serving, stir the chopped tomato and cucumber into the remaining half of the yogurt mixture. Cover and chill till serving time.

▲ In a large bowl combine the desired vegetables. Lightly spray vegetables with nonstick spray coating, tossing to coat. Stir in remaining oregano. Set aside.

▲ Drain pork. Alternately thread pork and vegetables onto twelve 6-inch-long skewers. Grill kabobs on an uncovered grill directly over *medium* coals for 12 to 14 minutes or till pork is tender and juices run clear, turning once halfway through grilling. Serve kabobs with sauce. Makes 6 servings.

Nutrition Facts per serving: 207 calories, 8 g total fat (3 g saturated fat), 53 mg cholesterol, 97 mg sodium, 13 g carbohydrate, 2 g fiber, 22 g protein.
Daily Values: 3% vitamin A, 44% vitamin C, 14% calcium, 9% iron.

The yogurt in the chunky vegetable sauce adds vitamin D and calcium to this fresh-tasting main dish. Vitamin D helps the body absorb calcium, which helps build strong bones and teeth.

Pork Tenderloin with Corn Salsa

Corn adds color, potassium, and fiber to purchased salsa, spicing up this quick-and-easy main dish.

12 **ounces pork tenderloin**
2 **tablespoons all-purpose flour**
1 **teaspoon chili powder**
⅛ **teaspoon salt**
2 **teaspoons cooking oil**
1 **cup frozen loose-pack whole kernel corn**
½ **cup salsa**

▲ Cut pork crosswise into 8 pieces. Place each piece between 2 pieces of plastic wrap. Pound with the flat side of a meat mallet till ¼ inch thick.

▲ In a shallow dish stir together the flour, chili powder, and salt. Dip pork into flour mixture, coating both sides.

▲ In a large skillet cook pork in hot oil over medium heat for 8 to 10 minutes or till juices run clear, turning once.

▲ Meanwhile, for salsa, in a small saucepan stir together corn and salsa. Heat through. Serve salsa over steaks. Makes 4 servings.

Nutrition Facts per serving: 185 calories, 7 g total fat (1 g saturated fat), 60 mg cholesterol, 229 mg sodium, 13 g carbohydrate, 1 g fiber, 21 g protein.
Daily Values: 7% vitamin A, 18% vitamin C, 1% calcium, 11% iron.

Cooking Meat Right

Even the leanest cuts of meat have some separable fat that you can trim away with a sharp knife. The best methods for cooking meat the lean way are broiling, pan-broiling, grilling, poaching, or roasting. For the juiciest results, cook lean meats to no more than medium doneness (160° to 170°). Lean meats cooked past this temperature tend to dry out and lose their flavor.

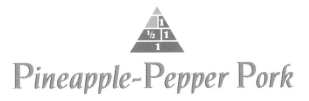

Pineapple-Pepper Pork

1   **8-ounce can pineapple chunks (juice pack)**
½   **teaspoon garlic salt**
¼   **teaspoon pepper**
12   **ounces boneless pork loin, cut into 4 slices**
2   **teaspoons cooking oil**
1   **medium green, red, and/or orange sweet pepper, cut into bite-size strips**
1   **small red onion, sliced and separated into rings**
2   **teaspoons cornstarch**
3   **cups hot cooked rice**

▲ Drain pineapple chunks, reserving juice. Add enough water to juice to equal ¾ cup. Set pineapple chunks and juice aside.

▲ Combine garlic salt and pepper; sprinkle over both sides of pork, pressing into surface of meat. Heat oil in a large nonstick skillet. Cook pork over medium heat for 10 to 12 minutes or till no pink remains and juices run clear, turning the meat over halfway through cooking time. Remove pork from skillet; keep warm.

▲ Add sweet pepper strips and onion rings to skillet. Cook and stir for 3 to 4 minutes or till crisp-tender. Stir cornstarch into reserved pineapple juices; add to vegetables in skillet. Cook and stir till thickened and bubbly. Cook and stir for 2 minutes more. Stir in pineapple chunks. Serve pineapple mixture over pork and hot cooked rice. Makes 4 servings.

Nutrition Facts per serving: 334 calories, 8 g total fat (2 g saturated fat), 38 mg cholesterol, 289 mg sodium, 48 g carbohydrate, 1 g fiber, 16 g protein.
Daily Values: 1% vitamin A, 35% vitamin C, 2% calcium, 14% iron.

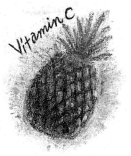

Pineapple and sweet peppers— what a perfect combination. Both are blessed with vitamin C, an antioxidant that has been linked with an increase in immune function and a decreased risk of cancer, heart disease, and cataracts.

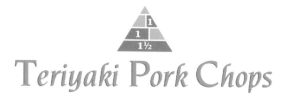

Teriyaki Pork Chops

Colorful vegetables top these chops. Carrots pack in the beta carotene, an important antioxidant that appears to help reduce the risk of cancer and heart disease.

⅛ teaspoon garlic salt
⅛ teaspoon ground ginger
⅛ teaspoon pepper
4 pork loin chops, cut ½ inch thick
   (about 1 pound total)
1 small red or green sweet pepper,
   cut into thin strips (¾ cup)
¾ cup coarsely shredded carrot
½ cup bias-sliced green onion
⅓ cup orange juice
3 tablespoon light teriyaki sauce
1 teaspoon cornstarch
¼ teaspoon bottled hot pepper
   sauce
3 cups hot cooked rice

▲ In a bowl combine garlic salt, ginger, and pepper. Trim fat from pork chops; sprinkle both sides of each chop with ginger mixture. Preheat a heavy 10-inch skillet over high heat till hot. Add chops; reduce heat to medium. Cook chops 8 to 10 minutes or till juices run clear, turning once. Remove from skillet; keep warm.

▲ Add sweet pepper, carrot, and green onion to the skillet. Cook over medium heat 2 to 3 minutes or till crisp-tender, stirring often. Combine orange juice, teriyaki sauce, cornstarch, and pepper sauce; add to vegetables. Cook and stir till thickened and bubbly; cook and stir 2 minutes more.

▲ Serve pork chops over hot cooked rice. Spoon the vegetable mixture atop chops. Makes 4 servings.

Nutrition Facts per serving: 332 calories, 8 g total fat (3 g saturated fat), 51 mg cholesterol, 313 mg sodium, 43 g carbohydrate, 1 g fiber, 20 g protein.
Daily Values: 102% vitamin A, 71% vitamin C, 2% calcium, 16% iron.

Easy Side Dish Ideas

Broccoli Salad: Combine 2½ cups broccoli slaw mix with 1 small chopped tomato; ¼ cup reduced-calorie buttermilk salad dressing; and 1 tablespoon snipped fresh basil or ½ teaspoon dried basil, crushed. Chill for up to 2 hours. Serve on a lettuce leaf. Makes 4 servings.

Snappy Green Beans: To 2 cups of cooked green beans, stir in 2 tablespoons chopped roasted red pepper; ¼ teaspoon dried marjoram, crushed; ¼ teaspoon dried basil, crushed; and a dash salt. Serves 4.

Cheesy Beans: Zip up a 16-ounce can pork and beans in tomato sauce. Add ½ cup of shredded reduced-fat cheddar cheese and 1 teaspoon chili powder. Serves 4.

Orange-Pecan Rice: When making rice, such as long grain, brown rice, or wild rice, use ½ orange juice and ½ chicken broth to make up the liquid. Stir in ¼ cup toasted pecans per 2 cups cooked rice just before serving.

Easy Curried Rice: Prepare 4 servings of long grain rice according to package directions, *except* add 1 teaspoon instant chicken bouillon granules, ½ teaspoon curry powder, and a dash pepper. Before serving, stir in ⅓ cup light raisins and ¼ cup chopped peanuts.

Healthful Baked Potato Topper: In a blender container blend till smooth ½ cup dry cottage cheese; 3 tablespoons skim milk; ¼ teaspoon salt; 1 tablespoon snipped fresh basil or ¼ teaspoon dried basil; ¼ teaspoon onion powder; and a dash pepper. Stir in ¼ cup plain nonfat yogurt. Makes enough for 4 potatoes.

Zesty Bean Salad: In a screw-top jar combine 3 tablespoons vinegar, 2 tablespoons molasses, 2 tablespoons salad oil, and 2 teaspoons Dijon-style mustard. In a bowl combine one 27-ounce can kidney beans, rinsed and drained; 2 stalks celery, sliced; and ¼ cup thinly sliced green onion. Pour dressing over beans; stir to coat. Chill 4 to 24 hours. Stir before serving. Serves 5.

Zucchini Salad: Shred a large zucchini; drain. Stir in ¼ cup reduced-fat dairy sour cream, ½ teaspoon Dijon-style mustard, and 1 teaspoon snipped fresh dill. Stir in 1 chopped tomato. Serve on lettuce leaves. Serves 4.

Buttermilk-Herb Potatoes: Prepare mashed potatoes as usual, *except* use buttermilk in place of milk and stir in 1 teaspoon snipped fresh herb, such as basil or sage, for each potato.

More Hot Mashed Potato Ideas
Add one of the following:
- ▲ Purchased pesto
  (about a spoonful per potato)
- ▲ Finely chopped roasted red pepper
  (about 1 spoonful per potato)
- ▲ Caraway seed
  (a dash per potato)
- ▲ Crumbled goat cheese
  (1 spoonful per potato)
- ▲ Chopped prosciutto
  (about 1 ounce per potato)
- ▲ Chopped fennel leaves
  (1 spoonful per potato)
- ▲ Lemon-pepper seasoning
  (⅛ teaspoon per potato)
- ▲ Nonfat ranch-style salad dressing
  (about 1 tablespoon per potato)

Lamb Chops with Orange-Mint Pesto

Herbs add flavor to foods without a lot of calories, sodium, or fat. For variety, substitute the spearmint in this recipe with apple mint or pineapple mint.

1 **cup lightly packed mint leaves (stems removed)***
½ **cup lightly packed parsley (stems removed)**
2 **tablespoons grated Parmesan cheese**
2 **tablespoons frozen orange juice concentrate, thawed**
1 **tablespoon olive oil or cooking oil**
⅛ **teaspoon salt**
⅛ **teaspoon pepper**
1 **clove garlic**
8 **lamb loin chops, cut ¾ inch thick (about 1¼ pound)**
Dash salt
Dash pepper

▲ For pesto, in a food processor bowl or blender container combine mint, parsley, Parmesan cheese, orange juice concentrate, oil, salt, pepper, and garlic. Cover and process or blend with several on-off turns till mixture is nearly smooth, scraping sides as necessary. Set aside *half* of the pesto. Cover and chill or freeze remaining pesto for later use.**

▲ Place lamb chops on the unheated rack of a broiler pan. Sprinkle lightly with salt and pepper. Broil 3 inches from the heat to desired doneness, turning once. (Allow 8 to 10 minutes for medium-rare and 10 to 12 minutes for medium.) Serve lamb chops with a dollop of pesto. Makes 4 servings.

*Note: If fresh mint is not available, substitute 1 cup more parsley and 1 teaspoon dried mint, crushed, for the fresh mint.

**Note: To freeze leftover pesto, place pesto in a freezer container; freeze for up to 3 months. Thaw overnight in refrigerator before using. Serve atop grilled meat or chicken or toss with hot cooked rice or pasta.

Nutrition Facts per serving with 2 tablespoons pesto: 217 calories, 11 g total fat (3 g saturated fat), 81 mg cholesterol, 170 mg sodium, 2 g carbohydrate, 0 g fiber, 27 g protein.
Daily Values: 5% vitamin A, 31% vitamin C, 4% calcium, 25% iron.

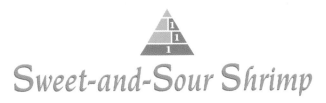

Sweet-and-Sour Shrimp

12 ounces fresh or frozen shrimp
    in shells
1 15½-ounce can pineapple chunks
    (juice-packed)
2 tablespoons vinegar
2 tablespoons light soy sauce
1 tablespoon cornstarch
1 tablespoon brown sugar
⅛ teaspoon ground red pepper
1 tablespoon cooking oil
1 teaspoon grated gingerroot
1 medium green or red sweet
    pepper, cut into 1-inch pieces
    (1 cup)
2 oranges, peeled and sectioned
2 cups hot cooked rice

▲ Thaw shrimp, if frozen. Peel and devein. Set aside.

▲ For sauce, drain pineapple chunks, reserving ½ *cup* juice. Stir the vinegar, soy sauce, cornstarch, brown sugar, and ground red pepper into reserved juice. Set sauce aside.

▲ Pour cooking oil into a wok or large skillet. (Add more oil as necessary during cooking.) Preheat over medium-high heat. Stir-fry gingerroot and sweet pepper in hot oil for 3 to 4 minutes or till crisp-tender. Remove from wok.

▲ Add shrimp to hot wok. Stir-fry for 2 to 3 minutes or till shrimp turn pink. Push shrimp from center of wok. Stir sauce; add to center of wok. Cook and stir till thickened and bubbly. Return sweet pepper to wok; add pineapple chunks. Stir to coat with sauce. Cook and stir 2 minutes more or till heated through. Stir in orange sections. Serve immediately over hot cooked rice. Makes 4 servings.

Nutrition Facts per serving: 297 calories, 5 g total fat (1 g saturated fat), 131 mg cholesterol, 417 mg sodium, 47 g carbohydrate, 1 g fiber, 18 g protein.
Daily Values: 7% vitamin A, 67% vitamin C, 5% calcium, 24% iron.

A small amount of brown sugar adds an additional touch of sweetness to this fruit-filled Oriental main dish. It's OK to use sugar in moderation in a healthful diet.

Shrimp and Sausage Jambalaya

Shrimp can be included in a heart-wise diet. Even though it does contain cholesterol, it is low in total fat and saturated fat.

12   ounces fresh or frozen shrimp
1   large onion, chopped (1 cup)
2   medium green sweet peppers, chopped
½   cup chopped celery
½   cup water
½   teaspoon dried thyme, crushed
¼   teaspoon crushed red pepper
⅛   teaspoon garlic powder
1   14½-ounce can low-sodium tomatoes, cut up
½   cup diced fully cooked smoked turkey sausage (about 2½ ounces)
4½   cups hot cooked rice

▲ Thaw shrimp, if frozen. Peel and devein. Set aside.

▲ In a large saucepan stir together the onion, green sweet pepper, celery, water, thyme, red pepper, and garlic powder. Bring to boiling. Reduce heat and simmer, covered, about 5 minutes or till the vegetables are tender. Stir in shrimp, *undrained* tomatoes, and turkey sausage.

▲ Return to boiling; reduce heat. Simmer, covered, for 2 to 3 minutes or till shrimp turn pink. Stir in rice and heat through. Makes 6 servings.

Nutrition Facts per serving: 253 calories, 2 g total fat (0 g saturated fat), 95 mg cholesterol, 226 mg sodium, 42 g carbohydrate, 2 g fiber, 16 g protein.
Daily Values: 9% vitamin A, 53% vitamin C, 6% calcium, 24% iron.

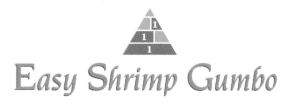

Easy Shrimp Gumbo

1 15-ounce can low-sodium tomato
    sauce
1 8-ounce jar chunky-style salsa
1 12-ounce package frozen, peeled,
    deveined shrimp, thawed
1 10-ounce package frozen whole
    okra
1 cup water
½ cup finely chopped fully cooked
    ham
1 teaspoon sugar
3 cups hot cooked rice
    Bottled hot pepper sauce
    (optional)

▲ In a large saucepan combine tomato sauce, salsa, shrimp, okra, water, ham, and sugar. Bring to boiling; reduce heat. Simmer, covered, about 5 minutes or till shrimp turn pink. Serve with rice. If desired, pass hot pepper sauce. Makes 6 servings.

Nutrition Facts per serving: 233 calories, 3 g total fat (0 g saturated fat), 93 mg cholesterol, 527 mg sodium, 37 g carbohydrate, 2 g fiber, 17 g protein.
Daily Values: 22% vitamin A, 70% vitamin C, 6% calcium, 26% iron.

Gumbo wouldn't be the same without okra, a vegetable that contributes fiber, calcium, niacin, and potassium to this dish.

Seafood Buying Guide

You don't have to be a fisherman to know a good fish when you see one. Here are a few tips to buying the freshest catch of the day:

Whole Fish. Look for eyes that are clear and bright, not sunken. The gills should be bright red or pink, the skin should be shiny and elastic, and the scales should be tight.

Fish Fillets and Steaks. Make sure the fish in the meat case is displayed on a bed of ice. The fish should have a mild smell, not a strong, fishy odor. Avoid fish that is dry around the edges.

Shrimp. Pick fresh shrimp that are moist and firm, with translucent flesh and a fresh aroma. Avoid shrimp with an ammonia-like smell.

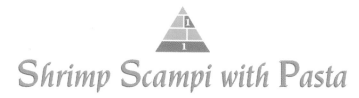

Shrimp Scampi with Pasta

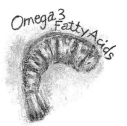
Omega 3 Fatty Acids

Shrimp and other shellfish or seafood contain omega-3 fatty acids, which have been shown to reduce the risk for heart disease and high blood pressure—all the more reason to enjoy the delicate flavors of this quick-to-fix dish.

12 ounces fresh or frozen shrimp
8 ounces spaghetti
2 tablespoons margarine or butter
½ cup thinly sliced green onion
4 cloves garlic, minced
1 tablespoon snipped fresh basil or
    1 teaspoon dried basil, crushed
⅓ cup chicken broth
3 tablespoons dry white wine or
    chicken broth
3 tablespoons lemon juice
2 teaspoons cornstarch
3 tablespoons snipped fresh
    parsley

▲ Thaw shrimp, if frozen. Peel and devein shrimp; set aside. Cook the pasta according to package directions. Drain.

▲ Meanwhile, in a large skillet heat margarine or butter over medium heat. Add shrimp, green onion, garlic, and basil. Cook over medium-high heat for 2 to 3 minutes or till shrimp turn pink, stirring frequently. Remove shrimp mixture with a slotted spoon.

▲ Stir together the chicken broth, wine, lemon juice, and cornstarch; add to skillet. Cook and stir till thickened and bubbly. Cook and stir for 1 minute more. Return shrimp mixture to skillet. Heat through. Stir in parsley. Spoon shrimp mixture over hot cooked pasta, tossing to coat. Makes 4 servings.

Nutrition Facts per serving: 368 calories, 8 g total fat (1 g saturated fat), 131 mg cholesterol, 286 mg sodium, 49 g carbohydrate, 1 g fiber, 23 g protein.
Daily Values: 16% vitamin A, 23% vitamin C, 4% calcium, 31% iron.

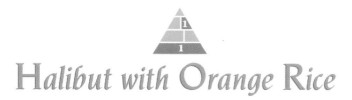

Halibut with Orange Rice

4 **fresh or frozen halibut or swordfish steaks, ¾ inch thick (1 to 1¼ pounds)**
¼ **cup orange juice**
1 **tablespoon brown sugar**
1 **tablespoon red wine vinegar**
Nonstick spray coating
Orange Rice

▲ Thaw fish, if frozen. Set aside.

▲ In a small skillet combine orange juice, brown sugar, and vinegar. Bring to boiling. Reduce heat and simmer, uncovered, for 5 to 6 minutes or till mixture becomes syrupy, stirring often. Remove from heat.

▲ Spray the unheated rack of a broiler pan with nonstick coating. Place fish on rack. Brush both sides of fish with 1 *tablespoon* of the juice mixture. Broil 4 inches from heat for 4 to 6 minutes per ½-inch thickness or till fish flakes easily when tested with a fork, turning halfway through cooking. Drizzle fish with remaining juice mixture just before serving. Serve with Orange Rice. Makes 4 servings.

Orange Rice: In a medium saucepan combine 2 cups *water*, ¼ cup thawed *orange juice concentrate*, and ¼ teaspoon *salt*. Bring to boiling; add 1 cup *long grain rice*. Reduce heat. Simmer, covered, about 20 minutes or till rice is tender. Stir in 3 tablespoons thinly sliced *green onion* or snipped *parsley*. Remove from heat. Fluff with a fork before serving.

Nutrition Facts per serving: 339 calories, 3 g total fat (0 g saturated fat), 36 mg cholesterol, 202 mg sodium, 48 g carbohydrate, 1 g fiber, 27 g protein.
Daily Values: 6% vitamin A, 59% vitamin C, 6% calcium, 21% iron.

Orange juice not only is a rich source of vitamin C, but also contains folic acid, a vitamin that helps prevent birth defects. You'll gain the nutritional benefits of orange juice from this light entrée and its easy accompaniment.

Swordfish with Mixed Fruit Salsa

With only 214 calories and 5 grams of fat per serving, this quick-to-fix dinner is a health bargain—and it's simply delicious, too. Add ½ cup cooked rice per person and you'll score one serving from the Pyramid Bread Group.

4 **fresh or frozen swordfish, shark, or halibut steaks, cut ¾ inch thick (1 to 1¼ pounds)**
Nonstick spray coating
2 **tablespoons lime juice**
¼ **teaspoon pepper**
1 **16-ounce can tropical fruit salad, drained and chopped**
2 **tablespoons lime juice**
2 **tablespoons thinly sliced green onion**
1 **fresh jalapeño pepper, seeded and chopped**

▲ Thaw fish, if frozen. Spray the unheated rack of a broiler pan with nonstick coating. Place fish on rack. Brush fish with the 2 tablespoons lime juice and sprinkle with pepper.

▲ Broil fish 4 inches from heat for 8 to 12 minutes or till fish just begins to flake easily when tested with a fork, turning once during cooking.

▲ Meanwhile, for salsa, in a medium mixing bowl stir together the drained fruit salad, the remaining lime juice, the green onion, and jalapeño pepper. Set aside. Top fish with salsa. Makes 4 servings.

Nutrition Facts per serving: 214 calories, 5 g total fat (1 g saturated fat), 45 mg cholesterol, 112 mg sodium, 19 g carbohydrate, 0 g fiber, 23 g protein.
Daily Values: 14% vitamin A, 54% vitamin C, 0% calcium, 6% iron.

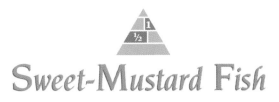

Sweet-Mustard Fish

1½ **pounds fresh or frozen fish fillets**
½ **cup salsa**
2 **tablespoons reduced-calorie mayonnaise dressing or salad dressing**
2 **tablespoons honey**
2 **tablespoons Dijon-style mustard or prepared mustard**
1 **large tomato, seeded and chopped**

▲ Thaw the fish, if frozen. Cut fish into 6 equal portions; place in a 13x9x2-inch baking pan. Bake the fish, uncovered, in a 450° oven for 4 to 6 minutes per ½-inch thickness or till fish just begins to flake easily when tested with a fork. Drain off any liquid.

▲ Meanwhile, stir together salsa, mayonnaise, honey, and mustard; spoon over drained fish. Return to oven for 2 to 3 minutes or till sauce is just heated through. Transfer to dinner plates; spoon any remaining sauce in baking pan over each serving. Sprinkle with the chopped tomato. Makes 6 servings.

Nutrition Facts per serving: 138 calories, 3 g total fat (0 g saturated fat), 43 mg cholesterol, 300 mg sodium, 9 g carbohydrate, 0 g fiber, 19 g protein.
Daily Values: 4% vitamin A, 17% vitamin C, 1% calcium, 4% iron.

With an extra kick from the salsa, this easy honey-mustard sauce is a perfect complement to fish. Chopped tomato adds freshness and vitamin C.

Hints for Cooking Fish

Just like any other meat, fresh fish should not be under-cooked or overcooked. Follow these visual guidelines when testing for doneness:
▲ Properly cooked fish is opaque, with milky, white juices. The flesh flakes easily with a fork.
▲ Undercooked fish is translucent, with clear juices. The flesh is firm and does not flake easily.
▲ Overcooked fish is opaque and dry. The flesh flakes into little pieces when tested with a fork.

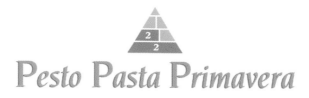

Pesto Pasta Primavera

Foods from the base section—the Bread Group—of the Pyramid, such as pasta, provide complex carbohydrates. Pasta comes in such a variety of flavors and shapes, you could serve a different type every day.

6   **ounces spaghetti**
1   **cup quartered baby pattypan squash, sliced zucchini, or sliced yellow summer squash**
1   **6-ounce package frozen pea pods**
1   **small red or yellow sweet pepper, chopped**
¼   **cup bias-sliced green onion**
¼   **cup Reduced-Fat Pesto (see recipe, page 46)**
¼   **cup chicken broth**
2   **tablespoons thinly shaved or finely shredded Parmesan cheese**

▲ Cook the pasta, uncovered, in boiling water for 7 minutes, stirring occasionally. Add vegetables; cook 3 minutes more. Drain pasta and vegetables in a colander. Return to hot pan. Add ¼ *cup* of the Reduced-Fat Pesto and the chicken broth, tossing till the pasta is well coated. Transfer to a serving platter; top with Parmesan cheese. Makes 4 servings.

Nutrition Facts per serving: 259 calories, 7 g total fat (2 g saturated fat), 4 mg cholesterol, 195 mg sodium, 40 g carbohydrate, 2 g fiber, 11 g protein.
Daily Values: 15% vitamin A, 75% vitamin C, 1% calcium, 20% iron.

For Good Measure

When you make pasta, do you ever end up with too much or too little for the number of people you're serving? Follow these guidelines so you'll end up with the right amount:
▲ 8 ounces uncooked small to medium pasta shapes (such as bow ties, elbow macaroni, or penne) = 4 cups cooked
▲ 8 ounces uncooked long pasta shapes (such as linguine, fettuccine, or spaghetti) = a 1½-inch in diameter bunch = 4 cups cooked
▲ 8 ounces uncooked egg noodles = 2½ cups cooked
Source: The National Pasta Association

Pasta with Artichokes and Basil

4 ounces tagliatelle, fusilli, or
   fettuccine, broken
1 9-ounce package frozen
   artichoke hearts, thawed
2 medium red or green sweet
   peppers, chopped
⅓ cup finely chopped onion
2 cloves garlic, minced
1 tablespoon olive oil
1 medium tomato, seeded and
   chopped
¼ cup snipped fresh basil or
   2 teaspoons dried basil,
   crushed
2 tablespoons grated Parmesan
   cheese

▲ Cook pasta in boiling lightly
salted water according to package
directions. Immediately drain. Return
pasta to pan; keep warm.

▲ Meanwhile, in a large skillet cook
and stir artichokes, sweet peppers,
onion, and garlic in hot oil over
medium-high heat about 5 minutes
or till vegetables are tender. Stir in
tomato and basil; cook and stir about
2 minutes more or till heated
through. Add artichoke mixture to
pasta. Toss gently to mix. Divide
pasta mixture among 3 dinner plates.
Sprinkle each serving with Parmesan
cheese. Makes 3 servings.

Nutrition Facts per serving: 278 calories, 7 g
total fat (2 g saturated fat), 3 mg cholesterol,
165 mg sodium, 46 g carbohydrate, 6 g fiber,
11 g protein.
Daily Values: 44% vitamin A, 171% vitamin C,
10% calcium, 21% iron.

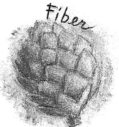

Fiber

*Artichoke hearts
are a calorie-
watcher's dream
come true with
only 37 calories
per ½-cup serving.
For lowest fat
content, choose
frozen rather than
oil-packed hearts,
which contain a lot
of fat.*

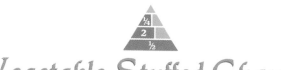

Vegetable-Stuffed Chayote

Chayote (cha-YOH-teh) is a summer squash with a funny name. But be adventurous and try it for a change. It's a good source of potassium, a necessary mineral which helps regulate your body's fluid balance.

2 medium chayote (8 ounces each)
1 cup sliced fresh mushrooms
½ cup chopped red sweet pepper
1 medium onion, chopped (½ cup)
1 clove garlic, minced
1 tablespoon margarine or butter
1½ cups soft whole grain bread crumbs, toasted (2 slices)
½ cup finely shredded Parmesan cheese (2 ounces)
1 beaten egg
2 tablespoons snipped cilantro or parsley
⅛ teaspoon salt
⅛ teaspoon pepper
¼ teaspoon instant vegetable or chicken bouillon granules
¼ cup water

▲ Halve chayote lengthwise. In a large saucepan place chayote halves in enough cold, salted water to cover. Bring to boiling; reduce heat. Cover and simmer for 12 to 15 minutes or till tender. Drain.

▲ When cool enough to handle, remove seeds. Scoop out and reserve pulp to within ¼ inch of skin. Invert shells; set aside to drain. Chop pulp; drain. If necessary, squeeze pulp between paper towels to remove excess liquid. Set aside.

▲ For stuffing, in a large skillet cook mushrooms, sweet pepper, onion, and garlic in hot margarine or butter till tender but not brown. Remove from heat. Stir in chayote pulp, bread crumbs, ⅓ cup of the Parmesan cheese, the egg, cilantro or parsley, salt, and pepper. Dissolve bouillon granules in water; stir into stuffing. Spoon stuffing into chayote shells.

▲ Place shells in a 2-quart-square baking dish. Bake, covered, in a 350° oven about 25 minutes or till heated through. Sprinkle with the remaining cheese. Bake for 3 to 5 minutes more or till cheese melts. Makes 4 servings.

Nutrition Facts per serving: 175 calories, 9 g total fat (3 g saturated fat), 63 mg cholesterol, 428 mg sodium, 16 g carbohydrate, 4 g fiber, 10 g protein.
Daily Values: 28% vitamin A, 51% vitamin C, 29% calcium, 11% iron.

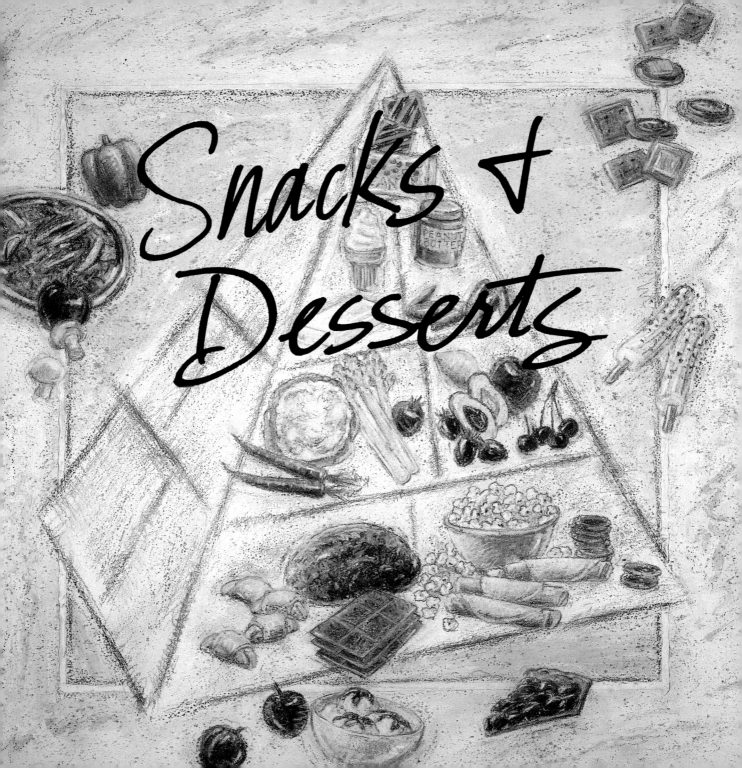

Snacks & Desserts

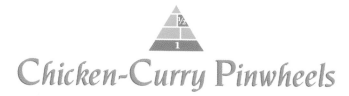

Chicken-Curry Pinwheels

Serve these healthful appetizers for a special get-together. The nuts contain vitamin E, an antioxidant, and their unsaturated fat content is easy on your heart.

¼ **cup plain low-fat yogurt**
1 **tablespoon tub fat-free cream cheese**
1 **tablespoon snipped chives or thinly sliced green onion**
½ **teaspoon curry powder**
⅛ **teaspoon salt**
¾ **cup finely chopped cooked chicken or turkey (4 ounces)**
2 **tablespoons chopped cashews or almonds**
6 **lettuce leaves**
6 **7-inch flour tortillas**

▲ In a small bowl stir together the yogurt and cream cheese. Stir in the chives or green onion, curry powder, and salt. Stir in chopped chicken or turkey and nuts. Place a lettuce leaf on each tortilla. Spread 2 *tablespoons* filling onto each. Roll up jelly-roll style; cut into slices. Serves 6.

Nutrition Facts per serving: 180 calories, 6 g total fat (1 g saturated fat), 19 mg cholesterol, 241 mg sodium, 22 g carbohydrate, 0 g fiber, 10 g protein.
Daily Values: 1% vitamin A, 1% vitamin C, 5% calcium, 11% iron.

This Nut's for You

Generally nuts are low in saturated fat, but all, except for chestnuts, are high in total fat and calories. Because nuts are such a concentrated source of fat and calories, keep your intake in check. Here are comparisons for 1 ounce of nuts:

Nut	Fat (g)	Calories
Pecans	19	190
Filberts or Hazelnuts	18	179
Walnuts	18	182
Almonds	15	167
Cashews	14	163
Peanuts	14	159

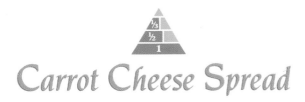

Carrot Cheese Spread

2 medium carrots, finely shredded
½ of an 8-ounce tub fat-free
   cream cheese
3 tablespoons grated Parmesan
   cheese
¼ teaspoon fines herbes or Italian
   seasoning, crushed
¼ cup Grape Nuts cereal
   Assorted whole-grain crackers

▲ In a small bowl stir together the carrots, cream cheese, Parmesan cheese, and fines herbes or Italian seasoning. Cover and chill at least 1 hour or overnight.

▲ Just before serving, slightly crush cereal. Shape cheese mixture into a 7-inch round; roll in crushed cereal to coat. Serve with crackers. Makes 10 servings (about 1¼ cups).

Nutrition facts per serving: 142 calories, 3 g total fat (1 g saturated fat), 27 mg cholesterol 354 mg sodium, 25 g carbohydrate, 2 g fiber, 6 g protein.
Daily Values: 74% vitamin A, 3% vitamin C, 73% calcium, 2% iron.

This cheese spread gets nutrition bonus points from carrots and crunchy cereal. Three to four crackers count toward one serving from the Bread Group.

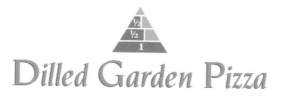

Dilled Garden Pizza

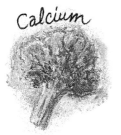

Calcium

You may have
thought that only
foods from the milk
group contained
calcium. But green
leafy vegetables,
such as spinach
and kale, and
broccoli also
contain calcium.
Calcium is needed
for bone and
teeth formation,
normal heart
rhythm, and
muscle contraction.

½ of an 8-ounce package
    reduced-fat cream cheese
    (Neufchâtel), softened
½ cup fat-free dairy sour cream
1 tablespoon finely chopped
    green onion
1½ teaspoons snipped fresh dill or
    ½ teaspoon dried dillweed
1 16-ounce package Boboli
    (12-inch Italian bread shell)
2 cups assorted chopped fresh
    vegetables (sweet peppers,
    broccoli, tomatoes, zucchini,
    jicama, cauliflower and/or
    shredded carrot)

▲ For dill spread, in a medium bowl
beat cream cheese, sour cream, green
onion, and dill with an electric mixer
till smooth. (If desired, cover and
chill up to 24 hours.)

▲ Spread the dill dip onto the bread
shell. Sprinkle with the assorted
vegetables. To serve, cut into wedges.
Makes 12 servings.

Nutrition Facts per serving: 140 calories, 5 g
total fat (1 g saturated fat), 9 mg cholesterol,
253 mg sodium, 19 g carbohydrate, 1 g fiber,
6 g protein.
Daily Values: 13% vitamin A, 29% vitamin C,
5% calcium, 6% iron.

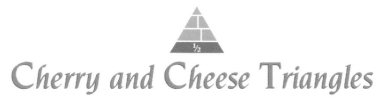

Cherry and Cheese Triangles

⅓ **cup dried cherries, snipped, or**
   mixed dried fruit bits
 1 **beaten egg**
 1 **cup low-fat ricotta cheese**
½ **cup sifted powdered sugar**
¼ **cup chopped toasted pecans or**
   walnuts
12 **sheets frozen phyllo dough**
   (18x12 inches), thawed
   Nonstick spray coating

▲ For filling, place dried cherries or fruit bits in a bowl. Pour enough boiling water over fruit to cover; let stand 10 minutes. Drain fruit. In a small mixing bowl beat egg, ricotta cheese, and powdered sugar till smooth. Stir in the fruit and nuts. Set mixture aside.

▲ Unfold phyllo dough. Cut sheets lengthwise in half. Place a half sheet of phyllo on a waxed-paper-lined surface. (Cover remaining sheets with a damp clean dishcloth; set aside.) Spray phyllo sheet lightly with nonstick coating; fold sheet in half lengthwise. Spray sheet lightly with more nonstick coating.

▲ Spoon a scant *tablespoon* of filling about 1 inch from one end of strip. Fold end over filling at a 45-degree angle. Continue folding to form a triangle that encloses the filling. Repeat with remaining phyllo dough and filling. Place triangles on an ungreased baking sheet. Spray the triangles with nonstick coating. Bake in a 375° oven about 15 minutes or till golden. Serve warm or cool. Makes 24 servings.

Nutrition Facts per serving: 60 calories, 2 g total fat (0 g saturated fat), 2 mg cholesterol, 55 mg sodium, 9 g carbohydrate, 0 g fiber, 2 g protein.
Daily Values: 1% vitamin A, 0% vitamin C, 1% calcium, 2% iron.

Dried fruits are concentrated sources of nutrition, but just a few add up to a lot of calories. By all means, enjoy them, but limit them to small quantities.

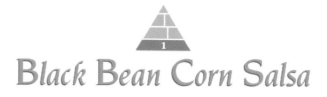

Black Bean Corn Salsa

Beans are higher in protein than any other plant food, but they lack the cholesterol and saturated fat found in meat products. Serve them in this salsa for a heart-healthy appetizer.

⅔ cup corn relish
½ of a 15-ounce can black beans, drained and rinsed (about ¾ cup)
¼ cup thinly sliced radishes
1½ teaspoons lime juice
¼ teaspoon ground cumin
Baked Tortilla Chips

▲ In a bowl stir together the relish, beans, radishes, lime juice, and cumin. Let mixture stand, covered, for 30 minutes. Serve with tortilla chips. Makes 12 servings.

Baked Tortilla Chips: Lightly spray eight 7-inch *corn tortillas* with *nonstick spray coating.* If desired, sprinkle lightly with *onion powder.* Cut each tortilla into 1-inch-wide strips. Spread strips in a single layer on a baking sheet. (You'll need to bake chips in batches.) Bake in a 350° oven for 10 to 12 minutes or till crisp. To store, place chips in an airtight container for up to 1 week.

Nutrition Facts per serving: 89 calories, 1 g total fat (0 g saturated fat), 0 mg cholesterol, 141 mg sodium, 20 g carbohydrate, 1 g fiber, 2 g protein.
Daily Values: 0% vitamin A, 1% vitamin C, 0% calcium, 2% iron.

Pita Crisps with Strawberry Spread

4 **large pita bread rounds**
Nonstick spray coating
½ **to ¾ teaspoon ground cinnamon**
1 **8-ounce tub fat-free cream cheese with strawberries**
1 **teaspoon finely shredded orange peel**
1 **tablespoon orange juice**
Fresh sliced strawberries (optional)

▲ Split pita bread rounds in half horizontally. Lightly spray the cut side of each pita bread half with nonstick coating. Sprinkle lightly with cinnamon. Cut each pita half into 6 wedges. Spread wedges in a single layer on a baking sheet. (You'll need to bake wedges in batches.) Bake wedges in a 350° oven for 10 to 12 minutes or till crisp. (To store the chips, place chips in an airtight container for up to 1 week.)

▲ For strawberry spread, in a small bowl stir together the cream cheese, orange peel, and orange juice. Serve with crisps. Makes 8 servings.

Nutrition Facts per serving: 125 calories, 0 g total fat (0 g saturated fat), 4 mg cholesterol, 161 mg sodium, 24 g carbohydrate, 0 g fiber, 7 g protein.
Daily Values: 10% vitamin A, 2% vitamin C, 10% calcium, 5% iron.

With more fat-free products available on the market today, it's easier than ever to cut fat from your diet. The strawberry cream-cheese product lets you enjoy this elegant dessert without guilt.

Easy Snack & Dessert Ideas

Yogurt Pops: Combine 1 cup unsweetened pineapple juice, one 8-ounce carton strawberry low-fat yogurt, and 3 tablespoons powdered sugar. Divide among 6 to 8 (3-ounce) paper cups. Insert wooden sticks and freeze till firm. Makes 6 to 8 servings.

Potato Fries: Cut 2 medium baking potatoes into 8 wedges. Stir ¼ teaspoon seasoned salt and ⅛ teaspoon pepper into 1 tablespoon melted margarine. Brush mixture onto wedges. Place wedges on a baking sheet sprayed with nonstick spray coating. Bake in a 450° oven for 30 to 35 minutes or till tender but crispy, turning once. Serve with nonfat ranch salad dressing. Serves 2.

Ricotta English Muffins: Combine ¾ cup low-fat ricotta cheese, ¼ teaspoon finely shredded lime peel, 2 teaspoons lime juice, 1 tablespoon sugar, and ⅛ teaspoon ground nutmeg. Spread onto toasted, split whole wheat English muffin halves. Top with sliced fruit, such as strawberries, kiwi fruit, or peaches. Serves 4.

Ice Cream Sandwiches: Spread ½ teaspoon red raspberry spreadable fruit onto each of 4 chocolate wafer cookies. Place about 2 tablespoons strawberry frozen yogurt on each of 4 more chocolate wafer cookies. Place cookies with raspberry spread (raspberry-side down) atop yogurt, pressing down slightly. Wrap and freeze at least 4 hours or till firm. Serves 4.

Pizza Snacks: Combine ¼ cup low-fat ricotta cheese and ¼ teaspoon dried Italian seasoning, crushed; spread onto 8 crispy rye crackers. Sprinkle with 2 tablespoons shredded reduced-fat mozzarella cheese and 2 tablespoons grated Parmesan cheese. Slice 4 cherry tomatoes; arrange slices atop each cracker. Bake in a 350° oven for 5 to 7 minutes or till cheese melts. Serve at once. Serves 4.

Creamy Lemon Dip: Combine one 8-ounce carton lemon low-fat yogurt and one 4½-ounce container-reduced-calorie vanilla pudding. Serve with assorted cut-up fresh fruit.

Parmesan Bagels: Combine 3 tablespoons nonfat mayonnaise dressing or salad dressing, 1 tablespoon grated Parmesan cheese, and 1 tablespoon snipped fresh basil or chives. Spread evenly onto 4 split whole wheat bagel halves. Broil bagels 3 to 4 inches from heat for 2 to 3 minutes or till toasted. Serves 4.

Chocolate Baked Pears: Place 2 cored, halved, and peeled pears, cut side up, in a 9-inch pie plate. Stir together 1 tablespoon lemon juice and 1 teaspoon vanilla or ½ teaspoon almond extract; brush onto pears. Bake pears, covered, in a 375° oven for 30 to 35 minutes or till tender. Uncover pears and sprinkle pear halves with 2 tablespoons miniature semisweet chocolate pieces. Serve pears at once. Serves 4.

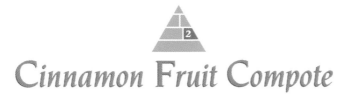

Cinnamon Fruit Compote

¾ cup white grape juice
1 tablespoon sugar
2 inches stick cinnamon
2 whole nutmegs
1 teaspoon finely shredded
      orange peel
1 cup strawberries, halved
2 medium nectarines, pitted and
      sliced
1 cup seedless green grapes
1 10½-ounce can mandarin orange
      sections (juice-packed),
      drained

▲ In a small saucepan combine grape juice, sugar, stick cinnamon, whole nutmegs, and orange peel. Cook and stir constantly over medium heat till sugar dissolves. Bring to boiling; reduce heat. Simmer, covered, for 5 minutes. Remove from heat. Cool 15 minutes. Remove cinnamon and whole nutmegs.

▲ Meanwhile, in a large bowl layer *half* of the strawberries and all of the nectarines, grapes, and orange sections. Top with the remaining strawberries. Cover and chill till serving time or up to 4 hours. To serve, pour juice mixture over fruit. Makes 8 servings.

Nutrition Facts per serving: 72 calories, 0 g total fat (0 g saturated fat), 0 mg cholesterol, 4 mg sodium, 18 g carbohydrate, 1 g fiber, 1 g protein.
Daily Values: 30% vitamin C.

For the greatest nutritional value, select grape juice that is 100% pure juice. If it's labeled "drink," it probably contains little fruit juice and lots of added sugar.

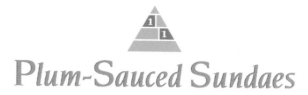

Plum-Sauced Sundaes

Spectacular desserts don't have to be sinful. This elegant sauce, served over ice cream, provides a serving from both the Fruit and Milk Groups.

¼ **cup sugar**
1 **teaspoon cornstarch**
5 **or 6 medium plums, pitted and sliced (2½ cups)**
2 **tablespoons water**
4 **cups vanilla low-fat or light ice cream**

▲ In a medium saucepan combine the sugar and cornstarch. Stir in the sliced plums and water. Bring to boiling, stirring occasionally. Reduce heat. Simmer sauce, covered, for 6 to 8 minutes or till of desired consistency.

▲ Cool the sauce slightly. Serve warm sauce over vanilla ice cream. Makes 8 (½-cup) servings.

Nutrition Facts per serving: 140 calories, 3 g total fat (2 g saturated fat), 9 mg cholesterol, 56 mg sodium, 27 g carbohydrate, 1 g fiber, 3 g protein.
Daily Values: 4% vitamin A, 7% vitamin C, 7% calcium, 0% iron.

We All Scream for Ice Cream

Ice cream is luscious. But many brands gobble up your fat intake for the day in just a few scoops. Ice cream is made from whole milk and cream, so it is generally high in saturated fat and cholesterol, too. But if you look for other frozen desserts that are low in saturated fat and total fat, you can enjoy desserts like the one here. Look for low-fat frozen yogurt, low-fat frozen dairy desserts, fruit ices, sorbet, frozen fruit juice bars, and low-fat ice cream. If you choose higher-fat varieties, eat just a small amount.

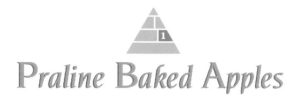

Praline Baked Apples

½ cup apple juice

⅛ teaspoon ground cinnamon

4 small red cooking apples

¼ cup coarsely chopped pecans or walnuts

¼ cup packed brown sugar

⅛ teaspoon ground cinnamon

Vanilla low-fat yogurt or low-fat ice cream (optional)

▲ In a small bowl combine apple juice and the ⅛ teaspoon cinnamon. Divide mixture among four 6-ounce custard cups. Core apples; remove peel from the top one-third of each apple. Cut apples into eighths, cutting to, but not completely through, the bottom. Place apples in prepared custard cups.

▲ Place custard cups on a shallow baking pan. Combine the pecans or walnuts, brown sugar, and remaining ⅛ teaspoon cinnamon. Sprinkle over the prepared apples. Bake, covered, in a 350° oven for 30 to 40 minutes or till apples are tender.

▲ To serve, dollop with yogurt or ice cream, if desired. Makes 4 servings.

Nutrition Facts per serving: 183 calories, 5 g total fat (0 g saturated fat), 0 mg cholesterol, 5 mg sodium, 37 g carbohydrate, 4 g fiber, 1 g protein.
Daily Values: 0% vitamin A, 13% vitamin C, 2% calcium, 5% iron.

Does dessert have a place in a healthy diet? Absolutely—especially when fruit is the star ingredient. The apples in this harvest-time favorite provide plenty of fiber. But be sure to leave the skin on for the most fiber benefit.

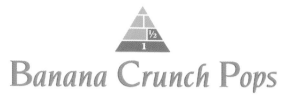

Banana Crunch Pops

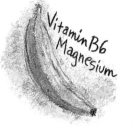

Bananas win praise for potassium, but just one also covers almost half of your vitamin B$_6$ requirements for the day. Replenish your B$_6$ daily to help prevent depression and strengthen your immune response.

1 **8-ounce carton nonfat yogurt (any flavor)**
¼ **teaspoon ground cinnamon**
6 **wooden sticks**
3 **bananas, peeled and cut in half crosswise**
1½ **cups low-fat granola or crisp rice cereal**

▲ Place yogurt in a shallow dish; stir in cinnamon. Insert a wooden stick into each banana piece. Roll banana pieces in the yogurt, covering the entire piece of banana. Place the cereal in a small, shallow dish. Roll the banana pieces in the cereal and place banana pieces on a waxed-paper-lined baking sheet. Place in the freezer.

▲ When frozen, wrap each banana pop in freezer wrap and label. Store pops in freezer. Let stand at room temperature for 10 minutes before serving. Makes 6 servings.

Nutrition Facts per pop: 156 calories, 2 g total fat (0 g saturated fat), 1 mg cholesterol, 56 mg sodium, 34 g carbohydrate, 3 g fiber, 4 g protein.
Daily Values: 12% vitamin A, 9% vitamin C, 7% calcium, 9% iron.

Metric Cooking Hints

By making a few conversions, cooks in Australia, Canada, and the United Kingdom can use the recipes in Better Homes and Gardens® *Eating Well with the Food Guide Pyramid* with confidence. The charts on this page provide a guide for converting measurements from the U.S. customary system, which is used throughout this book, to the imperial and metric systems. There also is a conversion table for oven temperatures to accommodate the differences in oven calibrations.

Volume and Weight: Americans traditionally use cup measures for liquid and solid ingredients. The chart (*top right*) shows the approximate imperial and metric equivalents. If you are accustomed to weighing solid ingredients, here are some helpful approximate equivalents.
▲ 1 cup butter, caster sugar, or rice = 8 ounces = about 250 grams
▲ 1 cup flour = 4 ounces = about 125 grams
▲ 1 cup icing sugar = 5 ounces = about 150 grams
  Spoon measures are used for smaller amounts of ingredients. Although the size of the tablespoon varies slightly among countries, for practical purposes, and for recipes in this book, a straight substitution is all that's necessary.
  Measurements made using cups or spoons should always be level, unless stated otherwise.

Product Differences: Most of the ingredients called for in the recipes in this book are available in English-speaking countries. However, some are known by different names. Here are some common American ingredients and their possible counterparts:
▲ Sugar is granulated or caster sugar.
▲ Powdered sugar is icing sugar.
▲ All-purpose flour is plain household flour or white flour. When self-rising flour is used in place of all-purpose flour in a recipe that calls for leavening, omit the leavening agent (baking soda or baking powder) and salt.
▲ Light corn syrup is golden syrup.
▲ Cornstarch is cornflour.
▲ Baking soda is bicarbonate of soda.
▲ Vanilla is vanilla essence.

Useful Equivalents

⅛ teaspoon = 0.5 ml	⅔ cup = 5 fluid ounces = 150 ml
¼ teaspoon = 1 ml	¾ cup = 6 fluid ounces = 175 ml
½ teaspoon = 2 ml	1 cup = 8 fluid ounces = 250 ml
1 teaspoon = 5 ml	2 cups = 1 pint
¼ cup = 2 fluid ounces = 50 ml	2 pints = 1 litre
⅓ cup = 3 fluid ounces = 75 ml	½ inch = 1 centimetre
½ cup = 4 fluid ounces = 125 ml	1 inch = 2 centimetres

Baking Pan Sizes

American	Metric
8x1½-inch round baking pan	20x4-centimetre sandwich or cake tin
9x1½-inch round baking pan	23x3.5-centimetre sandwich or cake tin
11x7x1½-inch baking pan	28x18x4-centimetre baking pan
13x9x2-inch baking pan	32.5x23x5-centimetre baking pan
2-quart-rectangular baking dish	30x19x5-centimetre baking pan
15x10x2-inch baking pan	38x25.5x2.5-centimetre baking pan (Swiss roll tin)
9-inch pie plate	22x4- or 23x4-centimetre pie plate
7- or 8-inch springform pan	18- or 20-centimetre springform or loose-bottom cake tin
9x5x3-inch loaf pan	23x13x6-centimetre or 2-pound narrow loaf pan or paté tin
1½-quart casserole	1.5-litre casserole
2-quart casserole	2-litre casserole

Oven Temperature Equivalents

Fahrenheit Setting	Celsius Setting*	Gas
300°F	150°C	Gas Mark 2
325°F	160°C	Gas Mark 3
350°F	180°C	Gas Mark 4
375°F	190°C	Gas Mark 5
400°F	200°C	Gas Mark 6
425°F	220°C	Gas Mark 7
450°F	230°C	Gas Mark 8
Broil		Grill

*Electric and gas ovens may be calibrated using Celsius. However, increase the Celsius setting 10 to 20 degrees when cooking above 160°C with an electric oven. For convection or forced-air ovens (gas or electric), lower the temperature setting 10°C when cooking at all heat levels.

Index

Keep track of your daily nutrition needs by using the information we provide at the end of each recipe. We've analyzed the nutritional content of each recipe serving for you. When a recipe gives an ingredient substitution, we used the first choice in the analysis. If it makes a range of servings (such as 4 to 6), we used the smallest number. Ingredients listed as optional weren't included in the calculations.

Serving Sizes

Bread, Cereals, Rice, and Pasta

Generally:

1 slice of bread
½ hamburger or hot dog bun
½ english muffin or bagel
1 small roll, biscuit, or muffin (about 1 ounce each)
½ cup cooked cereal
1 ounce ready-to-eat cereal
½ cup cooked pasta or rice
5 to 6 small crackers (saltine size)
2 to 3 large crackers (graham cracker square size)

Specifically:

4-inch pita bread
3 medium hard bread sticks, about 4¾ inches long
9 animal crackers
¼ cup uncooked rolled oats
2 tablespoons uncooked grits or cream of wheat cereal
1 oz. uncooked pasta (¼ cup macaroni or ¾ cup noodles)
3 tablespoons uncooked rice (about ½ cup cooked)
2 tablespoons uncooked barley (about ½ cup cooked)
1 7-inch flour or corn tortilla
2 taco shells, corn
1 4-inch pancake
9 3-ring pretzels or 2 pretzel rods
1/16 of 2-layer cake

⅕ of 10-inch angel food cake
1/10 of 8-inch, 2-crust pie
4 small cookies
½ medium doughnut
½ large croissant
3 rice or popcorn cakes
2 cups popcorn
12 tortilla chips

Fruits

Generally:

A whole fruit (medium apple, banana, peach, or orange, or a small pear)
1 grapefruit half
1 melon wedge (¼ of a medium cantaloup or ⅛ of a medium honeydew)
¾ cup juice (100% juice)
½ cup berries, cherries, or grapes
½ cup cup-up fresh fruit
½ cup cooked or canned fruit
½ cup frozen fruit
¼ cup dried fruit

Specifically:

5 large strawberries
7 medium strawberries
50 blueberries
30 raspberries
11 cherries
12 grapes
1½ medium plums
2 medium apricots

1 medium avocado
7 melon balls
½ cup fruit salad, such as Waldorf
½ medium mango
¼ medium papaya
1 large kiwifruit
4 canned apricot halves with liquid
14 canned cherries with liquid
1½ canned peach halves with liquid
2 canned pear halves with liquid
2½ canned pineapple slices with liquid
3 canned plums with liquid
9 dried apricot halves
5 prunes

Vegetables

Generally:

½ cup cooked vegetables
½ cup chopped raw vegetables
1 cup leafy raw vegetables, such as lettuce or spinach
½ cup tomato or spaghetti sauce
¼ cup tomato paste
½ cup cooked dry beans (if not counted as a meat alternate)

Specifically:

¾ cup vegetable juice
1 cup bean soup
1 cup vegetable soup